One Hundred Days, One Hundred Nights

One Hundred Days, One Hundred Nights

A Caregiver's Journey through Cancer

Gloria Burola McSorley

ABOOKS
Alive Book Publishing

Additional copies may be ordered from the publisher for educational, business,
promotional or premium use. For information, contact ALIVE Book Publishing at:
alivebookpublishing.com, or call (925) 837-7303.

Book Design by Alex Johnson

ISBN 13
978-1-63132-016-3

ISBN 10
1631320165

Library of Congress Control Number: 2015943379

Library of Congress Cataloging-in-Publication Data is available upon request.

First Edition

Published in the United States of America by ALIVE Book Publishing
and ALIVE Publishing Group, imprints of Advanced Publishing LLC
3200 A Danville Blvd., Suite 204, Alamo, California 94507
alivebookpublishing.com

PRINTED IN THE UNITED STATES OF AMERICA

10 9 8 7 6 5 4 3 2 1

To Richard John McSorley

who has been my friend and constant companion,

as well as the love of my life, for these past nineteen years.

Thank you for all you have given me,

shared with me, and taught me.

You will never be forgotten.

You are, and always will be, my world.

Contents

Acknowledgments

I would like to thank all who have helped and supported us along this journey.

To all those dedicated people at *Kaiser Permanente Hospital* in Walnut Creek, California: *Dr. Basil Adad* of Head and Neck Surgery, who helped us every step of the way; *Dr. Eugene Chan*, who was so kind and gentle with the feeding tube; *Dr. Chunnan Liu* and *Dr. John Simmons* in Oncology and Chemotherapy; and all the wonderful nurses in Infusion.

To all the caring, devoted people at the *Mt. Diablo Radiation Oncology Cancer Center*, Concord, California: *Susan Rausch*, the front office clerk, who greeted us with a smile each day; *Dr. Sakthi Vadivel, Dr. Roland Zimmerman*, and *Dr. Michael Levine*, who were kind and caring; and nurse *Edward Octaviano*. Special thanks go to all those who were so tolerant, gentle, and patient with Dick: therapists *Amanda Briggs* and *Hernando Montero* in Primus and *Colette Mellady*, who made the mask; and very special thanks to *Jill Rossi*, who was able to see trouble before it began and became more than just a nurse to us.

To our *friends* who helped us survive along the way:

Kathy Oliver, for checking up on me and, more important, for being there when I needed a shoulder to cry on as well as for all the food she brought early in the morning.

Bob and *Marilyn Young*, for being the best friends ever to laugh and cry with, and for all the encouraging cards.

Sally Schubb, for always being able to count on for her food, flowers, candy, wine, and editing.

Sally Barnik, a wonderful friend who understood what I was going through, and for all the cards and the beautiful framed picture of us.

Gretchen Hoffman, for adding more drama to my life and making me laugh.

Has Beans' *Chris and Gene Ono,* for giving us a second home, refuge, and resting place.

Vern Peabody, who gave us understanding and comfort with a hand on my shoulder and offers to drive to radiation.

And a special big hug and appreciation to *Christy Diggins* for the flowers, Champagne, food, wine, gifts, and all the phone calls that needed to be made. I am forever grateful for the help with our wedding announcements and endless editing. Thanks for caring and checking in on us each day and, most important, thank you for a gentle shoulder to lean on at my worst times.

And most of all to our *family,* who gave us support and comfort: above all, a special thank-you to *Tammy Burola Blanchard* and *Robin Burola La Fleur,* two of the best daughters I could ever have. Thank you for everything you did and said, including a strong arm, heart, and soul to lean on to keep me going when I felt like falling.

My bounty is as boundless as the sea,
my love as deep;
the more I give to thee,
the more I have,
for both are infinite.

—William Shakespeare, *Romeo and Juliet,* Act II, Scene 2

Introduction

The *American Heritage Dictionary* defines a caregiver as an "individual, such as a physician, nurse, or social worker, who assists in the identification, prevention, or treatment of an illness or disability," or as an "individual, such as a parent, foster parent, or head of a household, who attends to the needs of a child or dependent adult."

All my life I have been a caregiver, and I wasn't even aware of it. As a little girl growing up in New York, I took care of my younger brother and sister. Whether they got into trouble or needed a hand held while crossing the street, I was there. At nineteen, when my father deserted us, I was the one who stepped up and took the responsibility of helping our family make ends meet. When I got married, moved to California, and had children of my own, I became the ultimate caregiver, as every mother is. Complete love and devotion were what I was all about. That was my world, one in which I was content. I couldn't imagine anything else.

Later in life, my mother became very ill, and the term *caregiver* took on a whole new meaning. Whether it was open-heart surgery, quadruple bypass surgery, valve replacement, glaucoma, cataracts, anemia, diabetes, or eventual leg amputation, I was there. Although I was a full-time wife and mother, schoolroom aide, and Girl Scouts leader, and had a full, active life in California, I was continually there by my mother's side in New York. There were times when I would spend three days in California, fly to New York for four days, and then return to California, only to repeat the trip the next week. (I was connected with the airlines, so the flights were free.) There were occasions when I didn't think I would find the strength, but in the end I did.

After my mother's leg was amputated, the doctors informed her that she should be content if she could walk across the kitchen to make a cup of coffee. I saw the look on her face and told her to give me a year to get her hiking on the Pacific Crest Trail. One year later, we were there. My mother always said I was the one who added an extra ten years to her life.

And now, once more, I have been faced with the challenge of being the caregiver. This time I know exactly what that means. It is a role I take on willingly with a vast amount of love and devotion. It is not an easy job, and my shoulders sometimes feel a heavy burden, but it is who and what I am. There is no question that this is what I will be for the rest of my life.

One Hundred Days, One Hundred Nights is about two average people, Dick McSorley and Gloria Burola. There is nothing special about either one of us. We are just two people who had a wonderful life together before our world collapsed around us.

I met Dick twenty years ago, and most of that time we lived together as husband and wife, although we never made it official. Right from the beginning he told me, "There are only fifty-two weekends in a year, and I want to spend them all with you." And that's what we did, nonstop. We did everything together—skiing in the winter near my house in South Lake Tahoe, California, and sailing on the San Francisco Bay in the summer near his home. In between we shared other passions, such as motorcycling, hiking, traveling, and all the other things that made our lives complete. It was a good world with no worries.

As an avid sailor and captain of his own boat, before his illness, Dick liked to be master of his universe and in total command. As an engineer in the business world, he was very competent at figuring out most problems. Rarely was there something he could not accomplish with enough time and per-severance. Even now, failure is not a word he accepts well. I love that about him. On the other side, I love even more his protec-tiveness and gentleness around me, and I know he will always be my pillar of strength. His profound love for me is everything.

We were both healthy. Dick, a nonsmoker, had never really been sick, and I was the same way. Illness was just not a part of our world, nor was it a part of any of our children's world. Neither one of us was prepared for that first call with the diagnosis of cancer, nor for the path before us—a path no one wants to go down.

One Hundred Days, One Hundred Nights is a book written with passion about that path: a journey through cancer and every-thing that happens with it—the havoc it creates, the process of coping, and the light at the end. It is a book about the highs and lows and all the emotions in between. It is a story of love and perseverance, hope and disappointment, sadness and joy. It is all that and more. It is my heart opened wide to share my world and my life as a caregiver. What started as the jotting down of random thoughts to help me get through each day became so much more. It became a way to cope and survive. And at the end of each day I tried to find a bright side—which wasn't always easy to do, but it helped me maintain a delicate balance. The world around me went on; I just learned to see it a little differ-ently. I became more sensitive to everything that touched me, and I appreciated all I had with greater depth. I learned the real meaning of family and friends and cherished all the good mem-ories and good times. I realized what love was truly about.

Thinking positively and finding the bright side of each day made me stronger. It diverted my negative thoughts, at least for a moment, into good and positive ones. I could have, no matter how briefly, some pleasure and peace. And sometimes that was all I needed—to be able to go forward and cope with all that was to come, to give the best I had to offer, and to appreciate everything that had gone on before. Sometimes, all I needed to survive was to look on the bright side.

And most important, I found that being a caregiver is a whole world unto itself and the most important role of my life. There is so much to understand—so much emotion and so much strength needed. I found that knowledge and strength along the way and learned much that has helped me deal better with cancer and being a caregiver. I share it with you and hope it might make the journey easier for anyone else who gets that first call.

—*Gloria Burola McSorley, Caregiver*

Part One

One Hundred Days, One Hundred Nights

March

March

3/1 Wednesday. Day 1

We wait for the news we do not want, news we know is coming, news no one should ever have to hear. Push it away, cover my ears, do whatever I have to so I don't have to hear it. But the call comes anyway. . . .

Earlier today the doctor called me looking for Dick. I said he was on his way home. The doctor wanted to know if I would be there too. I said yes, and my heart dropped. He wanted us both there together. I already knew the news. Two days earlier when the biopsy was done, I had mentioned throat cancer and the doctor had replied, "I have my suspicions." I knew. Now we wait for the phone call, and wait and wait. It seems like forever. Suddenly, time is the most important thing that matters to me. Time is too slow waiting for a call, and time is not enough if something is going to be really bad. Time, waiting and time.

The call finally comes. Dick talks to the doctor and gets the inevitable news. "Yes, Dick, you do have throat cancer." Dick shows little expression. They talk. I wish I could listen. I hear him ask why they can't just operate. I don't hear the answer. Dick looks pale and sad. They talk some more and set up a doctor's appointment next Wednesday and also an appointment for radiation and chemotherapy. There—I have finally heard the words. The words I never want to hear around me, words that to me represent pain and suffering, sickness and death. I don't want any harm to come to Dick. I can't bear to think anyone will hurt him. It will kill me to see him suffer. I must remember to take one day at a time—just one day, or it will be too much to bear. I must be strong for both of us now. Dick has always been my rock; now it is my time to be his. I will. There is no question. I will be there for him, to hold his hand, to run his errands, to cope, to share. I will be there for everything.

Dick gets off the phone and says "Shit" softly, quietly, and I hold his hand and tell him I will be there, and we will get through this. And without question I tell him how much I love him and that he is my world. Perhaps that is too much of a burden for him to bear.

His son and daughter call, and he talks to them. I call my children and cry—a lot. What can anyone say? What can anyone do? We will keep everyone informed. Good-bye. We all feel helpless. "Shit!" and I do not say it quietly.

It is a hard evening. We are both numb. What will tomorrow bring?

On the bright side, I saw some deer eating happily in our neighborhood. I wonder if they could ever have the problems humans face.

I Knew

I knew I was right. Months ago Dick had started feeling a little off. It began with a cold that would not leave and a sore throat. The doctor prescribed antibiotics and cough medicine. I knew something was wrong. I said so. I told Dick to go back to the doctor, because it was something more. I thought *Throat cancer.* I knew I was right.

When my mother was going to go on vacation with my brother to the beach she loved, I told her it was too soon after she was out of the hospital, and she was not ready. We fought, the only time in our lives, so sad. She went anyway . . . and died. I knew I was right.

When my daughter got married so young, I tried to tell her it was too soon. She wouldn't listen. Wasted years later, she finally got a divorce, so sad. I knew I was right.

I knew something would happen to us. We had been too lucky. All the years we had been together, we were so happy. We had each other, friendship, love, sharing, good times, and our health. We had it all. I would often tell Dick, but I don't think he really understood. I had learned from my mother's sickness that health was the most important thing anyone could have. I knew we were too lucky.

So many times I knew. I am always right. What good does it do? Death comes anyway. Who cares if I am right? No one listens, so sad. And now Dick and I face hard times, and I do not want to think of the future because I

might

just

know

I

am

right.

3/2 Thursday. Day 2

The sun did come up today. I see the traffic outside, like timber wolves rushing. The world goes on. We are just a small part of it. Tomorrow is now today—where do I start? I get up early with Dick. I want him to know I am here for him. He says good-bye and goes off to work to see if this will be his last day. He isn't sure. He hugs me and whispers, "Thank you." There is a world in those words. We both understand. "Good-bye, I'll call you later," he says and goes off into the world without me. I already feel I have let him down. I will not be there to comfort him if he has terrible thoughts today or if he hears more awful news. I know I have to let him lead his life, but I want so much to protect him, and there is so little I can do, at least right now.

I call my aunt in New York and give her the bad news. She says she will pray for us. I go online and look up throat cancer. I think I am sorry I did; I do not like the news. There is that word again, *news*—the news on TV, the news in the newspapers, and now this . . . all bad news. *Shit.*

I will spend today running errands and trying to sort out what we do from here on. I just don't want to hear any more bad news.

I call my girlfriend, Kathy, and ask her to come over after work. I rarely reach out, so she knows something is wrong. There is no question she will be here. Good friends are special. We have some wine and talk. There are tears in both our eyes. She will be around if I need her—for comfort, in presence, in touch, in soul. It helps. I just need to let some of what's inside me out. Where do I start? I am so lost. This is all so new . . . and unwanted.

Dick comes home and joins us. There is no mention of anything heavy. I am not sure if Dick wants to acknowledge all that will be happening, either for him or for me. I don't know if he is scared, so I give him his space. Kathy leaves, and we settle down into our nightly routine . . . except I stay so much closer to him now. I want to savor every moment and to be around him if he needs me.

On the bright side, the mourning doves came back again this year to check out the planter on our deck. At least they have a new beginning. Also, Kathy and I saw a rainbow out the window against Mount Diablo. She said this was a good sign. I do not believe in signs.

3/3 Friday. Day 3

It's Friday. Usually we are up at our cabin in the mountains near Lake Tahoe by this time. I haven't been in the Bay Area on a Friday for months. It is ski season, and that is where we should be—but not now. There is a big storm up there dumping two or three feet of snow as I write. Travel would be too dangerous and tiring tonight, and I am already exhausted. All the emotions that have gone through me today have left me feeling drained. First, I was up and positive: I can cope with anything! Next, I was frustrated with so many questions and the hospital staff for not being able to get us any answers. I was on the phone forever with them and still got nowhere. Then I got angry because I had made no progress; and finally I was depressed and scared. Scared for Dick and scared for me. *What will happen to us?*

I hurt but I try not to show it. At one low point today, I called my girlfriend Sally, a nurse. I wanted her to be able to help, to be able to tell me she knew many patients who had been diagnosed with throat cancer and they were all fine, to be able to tell me about some magical medicine that would work fast. I wanted to be reassured, to make me feel better, like a warm, fuzzy blanket around my fears. She had no answers. It was a shock to her, too. We cried together. She knows how close Dick and I are and could tell how scared I was. But then we were able to talk and finally laugh. She did help after all. I've heard laughter is the best medicine.

On the bright side, it hailed and rained in between the sun and clouds. It is unusual for this time of year in California, but so is throat cancer. I saw another rainbow, small and brief, but there. Would Kathy say it was a sign?

*Rain, rain, go away, come back again
some other day*

*. . . Cancer, cancer, go away and don't
come back . . . ever.*

3/4 Saturday. Day 4

Saturday morning arrives. I am awake early and just watch Dick sleep. I want to be able to relish every minute I have with him. The way he is now. I touch his hair I love so much. Everyone admires his full head of hair.

He stirs. "What are you doing?"

"Just loving you," I say. He drifts off to sleep again, and I get up.

The calls are beginning to come in as news gets out. Friends from Lake Tahoe call and say they will keep him in their prayers. I mention it to Dick and he says "uh" and goes back to his computer. There is a strange distance in him right now. He seems not to want to acknowledge what is happening. Do I try to get him to open up or just wait until next Wednesday, when we see the doctor and get the full brunt of it? I decide to wait. I will have to find a support group to help me learn how to deal with this for myself and to help Dick. I feel so lost. I know others have been down this road; I just need to find them. In the meantime, we are off to the mountains to tie up loose ends and see the children. I wonder how the weekend will go. I think it is going to be hard.

When we arrive at the cabin three hours later, Dick has a headache but still insists on plowing the driveway. He is so stubborn. It is as if he has decided he is invincible. Nothing is going to touch him. He won't let it—nothing—and at this point, maybe, not even me.

I let him rest, build a nice fire to keep him warm, and cook him a beautiful dinner. He is still not himself.

"Is your headache going away?" I ask.

"Yes," he answers. Big conversation.

Finally we talk. He tells me to stop "clucking." I tell him I don't know how. I took care of my mother for ten years—being her legs when she had one amputated, being her soul and sounding board when the rest was taken away from her. I say I am a mother and caregiver, and I don't know any other way but to help. It is me, the essence of me. There are tears in my eyes. Dick says he is fine; so much for that.

We discuss my legal ability to be there for him and I ask, "Do you want a power of attorney or should we get married? Or maybe you don't want to?" Dick replies he has been with me these nineteen years because he wants to and we should go to Carson City, Nevada, and get married. I suggest here in Lake Tahoe, but do we need a blood test? I will find out tomorrow when I talk to my daughters. He still isn't feeling well, so we drop the subject. Besides, I have had too much wine and I am getting emotional. Maybe this is the problem, I show emotion and feeling and he shows nothing. He keeps saying he is fine. I know he isn't. And

I

am

always

right.

On the bright side, I saw seven deer as we were leaving for Lake Tahoe. That was nice. Also, the snow in the mountains is so beautiful, like whipped marshmallow cream, so pure, so innocent. Why can't I be that way?

3/5 Sunday. Day 5

Going skiing is good for both of us. It will get us out of the house and give us a chance to focus on other things. The outdoors always makes me feel better anyway, and the weather is holding. Sunday is busy and crowded. The main lift to the top is broken. Dick and I decide to carry our skis and walk up the hill. (Whatever possessed us to do that? Maybe we both need to relieve some stress.) Halfway up Dick decides to ski down, while I continue the rest of the way. Why? To prove I can make it? To be alone with my thoughts? To find perfect snow on the other side? I'm not sure, but it feels good.

Later I feel guilty and decide to start back and join Dick at home. I see him skiing and we join up. Split-second timing or we would have missed each other. Coincidence or luck, same as when we met. Is it a good sign? We ski together and I see how well he is doing, like nothing is wrong. Maybe it isn't. Maybe it is all a bad dream. Going down a beautiful trail home, he looks so handsome. I say a silent prayer to keep him that way.

Dick's son stops over. "How are you doing?" he asks.

"Fine," Dick replies. Denial.

My daughters had planned a special dinner for Dick and his son to celebrate their birthdays. It is really to just get us all together and be safe. It turns out to be a wonderful evening, a beautiful place overlooking Lake Tahoe and upstairs in a private dining room. So special and so appreciated, but too expensive. Both families together—I couldn't have asked for anything more. Please let it stay this way.

On the bright side, it was a good day and I got to see beautiful, standing lenticular clouds.

3/6 Monday. Day 6

I still have a hard time sleeping. I am up at 6:00 A.M. and wait forever for Dick to wake up. He doesn't want to go skiing because it is snowing lightly, so we don't go. I am disappointed but whatever Dick wants, at this point, takes priority. I just want to be with him. He questions why I am hanging around. How do I tell him I just want to stay near in case he needs me—for comfort, for support, to protect him, like the sentry dove we watch in the yard? I finally leave to run errands. I seem to annoy him. It is hard. I just can't seem to win . . . but then cancer sometimes has few winners.

At least by the end of the day, I have written a poem that is my favorite of any I've written. It explains why I want to be near Dick. I will give it to him tomorrow as a birthday present.

On the bright side, the snow is pretty on the trees, making intricate lace patterns.

What do you want for your birthday?

You can give me a new body.

I can't give you that, so I will just have to make

the body you have as good as new.

3/7 Tuesday. Day 7

Dear Dick,

Happy birthday, happy 73rd maybe. I know today will not be your best birthday. I know you too well. You will shrug it off and say it doesn't matter. You will be thinking of other things.

I do not have much to give you today. There has been so much going on, and I have not been able to get to a store to shop for a present. I know you don't want anything that can be bought anyway. You don't need it and what you do want and need, I am not able to give you — no one can. The best I can do is to give you this poem, along with my heart. To me they are the greatest gifts to give anyway.

Happy birthday, Dick, I love you.

Sentry Dove

I will be here for you, every moment, every day, always.
Like the doves that fly into the yard each morning,
I will be constant.
Like the doves that walk with one foot in front of the other,
carefully, assuredly,
I will take this challenge the same way, one step at a time,
carefully and with purpose.
Like the lone sentry dove that sits above the flock as they feed,
guarding, protecting,
I will be your sentry dove and protect you from the world . . .
as much as I can.
I will be strong and unwavering.
I will be your eyes, ears, and voice when needed to warn you
of danger and protect you.
I will be your sentry dove, and like the doves,
I will be with you for life.

———————————

On the bright side, we had a great day skiing in the powder. In the evening, I took Dick to a comedy show for his birthday. No, I took him to the show to take his mind off tomorrow. Let tomorrow never come. Best of all, Dick told me he liked the poem and wants me to frame it. That was a lot for him to say. For me, it was everything.

Do Not Let Wednesday Come

Do not let Wednesday come.
Let today stay just as it is.
Today we are safe. There will be no news from the doctor.
Today is a good day. Skiing is great. The snow is perfect.
Dick is happy.
We are free in the fresh air and our thoughts are
only on good things.
We do not think about tomorrow or the day after.
There is only today.
Do not let Wednesday come.
Wednesday, please stay away.

3/8 Wednesday. Day 8

Once more back in Danville in the Bay Area, Wednesday came anyway, no matter how much I tried to stop it. It came like an erupting volcano—violent, mean, and destructive—as I knew it would.

Dick and I see the doctor today and get the bad news. Some good news—no, it is all bad news. Dick has stage 3 squamous cell carcinoma. It is very bad, very serious. I hate Wednesday. I hate today. The doctor tells us that operating is not an option at this time. The cancer is too advanced, too large, and has already spread to the lymph nodes. He also tells Dick he needs to have a feeding tube inserted before he starts chemotherapy and radiation because he will probably not be able to take in enough food orally. We will learn more when we see the radiation doctor next week. The outlook isn't good. He mentions that only 35 percent of people diagnosed with this type of cancer live more than five years. The process is terrible, too—painful, draining, sickening, awful. Where is the good news? Where? When I am always able to find something in each day that makes sense, where is it now? How much more can I cry? I am so drained. I am trying to be supportive and strong for Dick, but I am falling apart inside.

We return home quietly. What can I say? I try, "I love you very much." It doesn't seem to register. Maybe we are both numb.

On the bright side, the mountains were beautifully covered with snow from the last storm. I wish I were there.

3/9 Thursday. Day 9

We are going right back to Lake Tahoe today, even though the trip takes three hours. It is what Dick wants. It will be raining in the Bay Area all weekend anyway. First he wants to stop at Has Beans, his favorite coffee shop, have a latte and see familiar friends. It is good for him, a comfortable routine in a warm and safe place. A friend stops by who has already gone through the same cancer treatment process. Dick seems to open up—a little. I think there must be a bond among cancer patients. I am sure as we continue on this journey we will find them. As the friend leaves he lays a hand on my shoulder to show support and says, "Hang in there." I needed that. I needed to know there may be hope. I wonder what Dick is thinking. I hope the same thing.

The trip up to the mountains is good, like the other times we've come up to have fun. It is like leaving the evil behind us, as if up here all will be well and no sickness can follow us. It is as if every mile we drive, the further away from pain and suffering we will feel. And Dick drives fast, as if to show he can get away from all the bad even sooner. At least for today we are safe.

We don't have to have the other shoe drop until next week, when Dick will see the chemotherapy and radiation doctors. I will hate Tuesday also, but for now we are away and free.

On the bright side, the mountains are so beautiful. Another storm brought more whipped marshmallow cream snow. I love it here where the accumulation is measured in feet, not inches.

3/10 Friday. Day 10

The night has come and gone with little sleep. I wake, and everything comes flooding back like a slow tide ready to take away your favorite sand castle—the one that took so long to build, of which you were so proud, the one that was just perfect. The inevitable tide creeps back and takes it away all too soon. I just want some peace, not another day of *What if*, *What will be*, and *Why*. We are going skiing in hopes of pushing all of that away. I wonder if it ever works.

On the bright side, the powder today was the best it has been in years, and I even ventured into the trees. So new to me, just like this past week has been. A week of new things—but some of which I would rather not discover.

3/11 Saturday. Day 11

Another night has passed without much rest. I listen to Dick breathing abnormally, a constant reminder of the hidden agony inside him. I wake up often because of it, and I have a hard time going back to sleep. We are both beginning to look tired. I know it is important for us to keep up our strength, both to fight this disease and for each other.

The waiting is hardest. It is the inability to know exactly what lies ahead paired with the certainty that *it*, no matter what *it* is, will come.

This cancer is like a hurricane that has disrupted our lives. You always know hurricanes are around, but you never really think one will hit you. And then you get the news, it is coming—and you wait. You wait to find out how bad it will be, how strong, how wide a path, how destructive. They put numbers on hurricanes to say how terrible. They put numbers on cancer the same way: T2N2AM0. This is the number Dick's cancer has been given. I hate these numbers. You try to prepare for a hurricane by boarding up your home and taking in supplies. You try to think of everything you can do so it will destroy as little as possible and make it easier to deal with. You can even leave town.

We can't leave town. There is nowhere to go. The options are few. We will have to be positive and rearrange our lives to prepare for what is to come. And *it* is coming soon, with a vengeance and, like a hurricane, strong, powerful, and destructive. We will have to weather *it* because that is all we can do.

On the bright side, today was the best powder day I have ever had. I didn't want to come in, but Dick was cold and tired. Whatever he wanted was fine with me. He said I should stay out and ski. I answered, "I can ski anytime, I want to be with you," and we returned home. At least for a while, the rest of the world stayed away.

39

3/12 Sunday. Day 12

I wake up to snow falling outside—hard, heavy, and straight down, like the tears I cried all night. I kept trying to find a way to make this cancer all better, to make it go away, to ease the process Dick has to go through, to be able to say the right words, to find comfort—somewhere, anywhere. I could find no answers, only tears.

I cry silently at night when I am alone with my thoughts and Dick cannot see me. I need to be strong for him. Dick mentions he is going to argue with the doctor about putting in a feeding tube. For the first time I quarrel with him. I have heard too many stories about not getting a feeding tube inserted before chemotherapy and radiation and the problems that arose afterward. "No, this time you can't have it your way. You will need this now to help you live. You are going to have to start to listen to me. We are going to fight this together, and I am going to be strong for you," I say. And for the first time, Dick does not argue back. I think he is beginning to understand.

I decide to let Dick sleep. I continue writing.

Later Dick asks, "Why didn't you wake me?" I reply, "It is very cold outside and I thought you might like to sleep." I am motioned back to bed with that look in his eyes. We love and embrace each other and, for a short time, the rest of the world stays away. He holds me close in his arms and we both feel protected and safe. We know we have each other. We have a little peace. Then the phone rings.

A friend calls because he hasn't heard from us and is worried.

"Yes, all is not the best," I say and put Dick on the phone.

"No, I'm sick," he says and sugarcoats the rest of the conversation. He is still not ready to reach out.

We have a late breakfast and go skiing anyway. It is the latest we have gone out, but Dick wants to be on the mountain. Maybe it is his escape. It is still hard to know his feelings. We have the best day ever, unbelievable powder and fresh air. Run after run we ski hard, as if we can outpace all that is to come.

In the evening we have his son and grandson over for dinner, and for a while we all laugh, and it is as if nothing was ever wrong. Except for a slightly hoarse voice, Dick is like his old self. It is so good to see.

On the bright side, all things considered, this was a pretty good day.

See these arms?
They are for wrapping around you.

3/13 Monday. Day 13

It is already beginning. I do not believe in superstitions like black cats or the number thirteen but, just maybe, there is something to it. I hear the word *Wednesday*.

Today starts just like the ones before. I get up early and let Dick sleep because I think he doesn't want to go skiing. I am wrong. When Dick finally gets up and has a late breakfast, he decides he wants to go out. Off we go, very late but much needed, to escape for a few hours. It feels good and we both know it.

Finally it is time to pack up and drive back home to the Bay Area to face reality. The drive itself is quieter than usual. I think we both realize it is now time to "face the music" and we can no longer put off the inevitable.

Upon arriving back in Danville, I pick up the messages on the answering machine. First the hospital called to confirm Dick's appointment tomorrow. Then there are two calls to say he has been rescheduled for Wednesday instead. I really hate Wednesdays. The message explained that the doctor was sick and it was important for Dick to get in as soon as possible. Another patient had to be rescheduled to accommodate him. "Please call and confirm."

Dick goes crazy. He is upset that he had to drive three hours down to the Bay Area and could not have another day of skiing. He is angry with the hospital for not being able to contact him even though he has given them all the telephone numbers. He is still in denial.

I look him in the eye and give the anger right back. I tell him how hard it is to get an appointment and how they are doing the best they can. And I tell him, for the first time, that every minute is crucial, that this is important. He knows I'm serious and calms down. I can tell it is going to be a very long, hard road for both of us, and we haven't even heard the worst of it yet. I know I will hate Wednesday.

On the bright side, it was another good day on the mountain and we had each other.

Will You Listen Now?

You did not listen when I told you we were so lucky we found
each other.
You did not listen when I said we should be grateful for
all we have.
You did not listen when I said we should not take anything for
granted—especially our health, the most important of all.
You did not listen when I said
to take care of your "cold" and see a doctor.
You did not listen when your sore throat did not go away.
You did not listen when I told you all the cough drops were
not helping—it was something more . . .
and I thought throat cancer.
Time and time again, you did not listen.
Now time is running out.
Will you listen now?

3/14 Tuesday. Day 14

We wake up to a very rainy morning, like the heavens are crying with us. It is going to be a hard day waiting for tomorrow's doctor appointment. Wednesday. I hate Wednesdays. For today we will just have to go about our routine, getting errands done and catching up on business.

I call to confirm Dick's appointment and get a lot more information than I ever intended to get or can process correctly. The nurse I speak with is very nice but tells me more than I can comprehend at the time. She explains all about the feeding tube and how I may have to be taught to insert liquids into it. She talks about the doctors, not sugarcoating anything, but they are a team who works together; and she even mentions the word *hospice.*

I am drained, scared, devastated, faint, and instantly start to get a headache (which I never do). What is worse, this is just the beginning of the news we will hear tomorrow . . . and Dick doesn't have any idea. How do I tell him? How do I prepare him for what is to come? Do I let a stranger break it to him like a freight train out of control, hitting him head-on? Do I let him get the horrible lump at the bottom of his stomach like the one I feel right now? Do I try to comfort him before we get there tomorrow? Where are all the answers I need right now? I think I should at least try. I will let him lash out at me and get some of the anger he must feel off his chest. It is going to be such a hard day. Why can't it just go away and we go back to the wonderful life we had before?

Later I finally start to address some of what is to come with Dick. At first he says not to worry about it, that it is his problem. He's still holding everything in and showing little emotion. He wants to change the subject. He is still not really aware of what is about to happen. He has done nothing to ready himself for all he has to go through. He is still in denial. I understand, but that will not help him tomorrow. He needs to be somewhat prepared.

As a friend suggested, I start to open up to Dick, for both our sakes. I tell him he can hear some of this from me, the one who is closest to him, or from a stranger, maybe a good doctor but still a stranger. I explain a little of what is ahead, and as always, I tell him I will be with him forever. I say I'm scared and I don't want to see him hurt. I cry, tears streaming down my cheeks, but I cannot hold back my feelings any longer. I need to acknowledge that this cancer has affected me too and he needs to see that. We are in this together, and I will be there all the way. I think he is beginning to be aware, but maybe he is also trying to be strong for me. I am not sure. This time he is hard to read as he is a very proud, private man. I think tomorrow a lot will change.

We go out to dinner and at least I can breathe better. Some of the weight I have been carrying around these past weeks has been lifted. Dick does not eat his usual amount. He is still trying to lose weight. I think the weight of cancer he now carries around will not be lifted for a long, long time.

On the bright side, a friend came over so I could let some of my emotions out. It is a beautiful thing to have a friend. Thank you, Kathy.

47

3/15 Wednesday. Day 15

Today is Wednesday. No matter how much I tried to stop it, it came anyway. I hate today. I am up early again. This seems to be my new pattern. As soon as I wake up, I can't get back to sleep. All the reality I don't want to face comes flooding back to me. It is still raining. It is going to be a hard day, but we have to face it head-on.

At least at this moment, I feel better. Opening up last night to Kathy has made a difference. I feel stronger and more positive, and that will help at the doctor's office today. I have to keep my head clear so I can absorb everything we are going to hear. It is so easy to short-circuit when you get bad news and so difficult to process what you learn. We are going to get through this. I am ready. Off to the hospital we go.

No, I am not ready. No matter how prepared you might think you are, you are never prepared to hear the worst. There still must be hope. Where is that hope now? The second doctor we see today, who will be in charge of chemotherapy, says Dick does not have stage 3 cancer but stage 4. My heart drops. I am afraid to look at Dick. I don't know if it has registered with him how bad this news is.

The doctor goes on to say there may be a 40 percent chance of survival past five years. The cancer is at the top of the throat, and the problem with that, besides not being operable now, is that this cancer usually comes back. It comes back again! After all the shit Dick will have to go through, it will probably come back! It will return to haunt him and make his life miserable, to cause him pain and suffering again. I can't believe it when the doctor utters these words. Again, there is not much reaction from Dick.

We are given more information today than our brains can possibly absorb correctly. Everyone is nice and patient. We are told that everything will be explained several times because it is so hard to comprehend. They deal with this every day and realize how difficult a time it is for the patients and their families. Dick has his weight, height, and blood pressure taken. Then we meet with a pharmacist who explains about all the medicines Dick will have to take and their side effects. We are shown the infusion room, the section of the hospital where the chemotherapy will be administered. A dozen people seated in large recliner chairs are already undergoing the process. He will have to stay here for five to six hours for each chemo infusion. Dick finally shows emotion. He is not happy with the idea he will have to be here that long. It is scary. The lump in the bottom of my stomach returns. I feel ill, light-headed, scared, and wonder what Dick is feeling. He needs to feel and get some of what is inside him out. We are told the hospital will call us when all the appointments have been scheduled. Two hours later we pick up a urine-sample bottle and head home. Both of us are drained. The ride home is quiet. I feel numb.

The rest of the evening is subdued. I can't even talk, and Dick seems to feel the same way. Tomorrow is another day. Possibly it will be better. I have to have hope.

On the bright side . . . on the bright side, spring is beginning to arrive, and Dick and I have each other.

Cancer

Cancer has no respect.
Cancer knows no right or wrong.
Cancer invades anyone, anytime, anywhere, any way.
Cancer is undiscriminating and unforgiving.
Cancer affects the rich or poor, good or bad, young or old.
Cancer has no middle ground.
It is what it is—you have it or you don't.
No matter what kind of cancer, it devastates.
Cancer is a miserable villain,
which causes pain and disrupts lives.
And like all villains, it must be destroyed.
Cancer cannot win this war.

3/16 Thursday. Day 16

Today is another day. We have been told many times to take it one day at a time, and we are. This is another day. We have the usual morning of a stop at Has Beans and run some errands.

Maybe *usual* is not the right word. What is usual these days? Cancer in my life is not usual. This is entirely foreign to me, and I do not like it. Most of my life I loved to do extraordinary things and to be different. I loved to take chances, explore the unknown, and live on the edge. *Usual* was not in my world. Everything I do now I look at with a different perspective. Is it really that important? Do I need to address it right at this moment? Does it really matter? What are my real priorities? The answer is always the same. My only priority is taking care of Dick and getting him well.

We pack up the car and head up to the mountains for the weekend for a few days away in the fresh air, skiing and seeing family. Over three feet of snow fell in the past twenty-four hours, and the skiing will be great. I realize it may also be the last time. The doctor has already warned Dick that once treatments start he will not be able to be far away from the hospital in case of fever and other complications. This is really serious. I hope Dick understands. No matter how unrealistic it seems, at least for now, going to the mountains is our escape. It is also something we would usually do. At least, for the moment, we are normal.

On the bright side, Dick and I are in this together. He will never be alone.

3/17 Friday. Day 17

Another day and one step at a time. Waking up to a beautiful world outside my window helps me feel better. The snowstorm has left the earth pure and simple and, most of all, peaceful. That is all I want now, some peace. Every waking moment is filled with torment. *What if? What will be? What could have been?* Sometimes to the point I think I will explode. Doctor appointments, schedules, phone calls, processing information I do not want to hear. I just need some peace.

I want to go skiing so badly this morning. The conditions are perfect, powder snow and light skies. I can't wait for Dick to get up, excited to be able to get out and away from the problems we have to face, if even for just a little while, to be free and happy. Dick finally gets up and says he doesn't want to go. That ends that.

Instead, today is filled with errands and responsibilities—making arrangements to close up the house, listing the condo I bought last fall for sale, sorting out projects, and generally trying to get things on track. It is St. Patrick's Day, a day we don't really celebrate. Actually, we end up doing something special today. We get a marriage license. Funny, it took something like cancer in our lives for us to finally do this after nineteen years. We had talked many times about getting married but just never seemed to get around to it. There was always something more important that had to come first—children got married, vacations were planned, work got in the way. There simply never seemed to be the right moment or a pressing need. We both knew how we felt, and no piece of paper was really going to make a difference. Someday . . . it was always someday. We just never got around to it, though we knew someday would eventually come.

On the bright side, I know Dick really loves me.

I Wonder

I wake up early in wonder at the view before me.
It has been snowing all night, silently.
The world outside is tranquil and still.
The trees are covered delicately, like tatted lace.
Nothing is moving, as if time itself has stopped.
I wish time could stop for me.
I marvel how God can create such beauty.
Yet I wonder how that same God
can let there be so much pain.
So begins another day.

3/18 Saturday. Day 18

Finally, we are going skiing. It will be more crowded today, but at least we are getting out. I can't wait. It is very cold, with snow showers, and the visibility isn't the best, but it feels wonderful anyway. We ski a lot of our favorite runs, and for the first time I notice a change in Dick's skiing. He is not quite as fast, and a few times I even have to wait for him. Maybe the light is flat and hard to see ahead. Also, I don't think either one of us is at our best. We are not getting enough sleep, and we have that constant cancer cloud over our heads.

We finally decide to start back. As we round a corner, Dick is down. I can't believe it. He never falls.

"What happened?" I ask.

"I don't know, maybe a mogul," he answers. He picks himself up and we ski on.

And then something does happen. On the way down in the tram, Dick all of a sudden says, "I don't feel well." He never says that. He never admits he is weak, sick, or unable to do anything. He is a rock and will not allow himself to be anything less. He looks scared for the first time. I hold his arm in case he starts to faint. A friend in the tram offers to get his car and drive us home, even though we live across the street. Dick agrees. Now I know he isn't himself. Dick never accepts help from anyone.

Back at the house we discuss what has just happened and what might have brought it on. I say maybe the high altitude and not being able to take in as much air as usual could have made him light-headed, or maybe he isn't getting enough sleep. Whatever it is, for the first time I see it in Dick's eyes. He is afraid. Cancer is beginning to torment his mind as well as his body. We let it pass as family is coming over this evening, for both comfort and love.

Later at dinner my daughters bring up the subject of us getting married. They keep saying we need to get married now while the families are all together and before Dick starts treatment and doesn't feel well. The problem is that we are leaving Monday morning for the Bay Area and might not return. Also, in three days Dick's son is going out of the country on vacation. How can it be done? My children say getting married tomorrow is the only answer. I reply that less than twenty-four hours is too little time and I can't cope with it right now. I can't see how it can take place so soon. They respond by saying they can take care of everything. The subject is then dropped as they both have exciting news to share. Both my daughters, Tammy and Robin, announce they are pregnant, have the same doctor, and are due about the same time! It is equally astonishing and delightful, and it will give me something, besides this cancer, to focus on. I go to bed that night feeling better but not knowing what Sunday will bring.

On the bright side, it was great to have both the children and their husbands come to dinner. It was especially wonderful since they announced their pregnancies. All in all, it was quite a memorable day.

3/19 Sunday. Day 19

I cannot believe what is actually happening to me right now. I am so filled with emotions I am ready to burst. We are getting married today! After the subject was brought up last night, my daughters had said they could take care of everything, and they did! God bless children. I have such good ones. I know I am very lucky. I had gone to bed last night not knowing what Sunday would bring, and now it is here. I still can't believe it, so little time, and so much emotion.

Tammy calls us at 8:00 A.M. She couldn't wait any longer. "Congratulations, Mom, you are getting married today! Robin and I are taking care of everything. I will call you later." I'm not sure I heard right. And so the day begins. I do laundry, dishes, and generally get the house ready to close up. After many phone calls back and forth, everything starts to fall into place. With each call there is more excitement in Tammy's voice.

"Where do you want to get married, still on top of the mountain? We have arranged for the gondola to take us all up after everyone else has come down for the day."

"I would like that, but the weather may not cooperate, I think it is going to snow."

"We'll see. What kind of flowers do you want?"

"Flowers, I can't even think about anything. I think I am numb at the moment."

"What about rings? Do you have them?"

"No, I don't even know where to go."

"I'll call you back with the information."

"By the way, what time are we getting married?"

"Oh," she says, laughing, "Five P.M. today. Don't worry, Robin and I will take care of everything. 'Bye, Mom." And so the day continues.

Dick and I run errands and go to pick out our wedding

bands. He holds my hand tight. We are ready—too bad the weather isn't. We decide at 3:30 to cancel having the wedding at the top of the mountain because the snow is coming in and Dick would be too cold.

"Where else do you want to have it?" Tammy calls from the car.

"I don't know," I say. "We can just have it at the house."

"I'll call you back," she replies and is gone.

We were all supposed to meet at 4:45 P.M. to go up the gondola; it is already 4:00. We still have to notify Dick's son and family of the change in plans.

Tammy finally calls back: "Mom, I got a place. You are getting married by the lake in a private room with a fireplace so it will be warm for Richard." (They call him Richard.) She gives us directions and says with a bounce in her voice, "See you there at 4:45 P.M."

And so we get married! It is wonderful. My granddaughter is even my flower girl, snow boots and all. I recite the "Sentry Dove" poem I had given Dick (page 34) and he speaks about this being the second-best day of his life (the first one being when he met me).

On the bright side, it was indeed a very, very bright day!

57

Our Wedding Ceremony

Almost twenty years ago, on May 28, 1987, who knew love would find you both on a flight to Europe? With that love came a feeling so powerful and so pure, it has been an invisible lifeline between the two of you.

As you know, love is demonstrated when each partner puts their loved one's happiness before their own. And in true love the permanent good of the partnership is far more important than any temporary pleasures.

True love manifests itself through loyalty, honesty, communication, and faith in each other's integrity.

Believe in love—believe in the love you have for each other And most important as you journey through life, be very gentle with each other's heart.

Richard and Gloria, do you stand before me today to vow your loyalty and devotion to one another?

Richard, in taking Gloria to be your lawfully wedded wife, do you promise to love, honor, and cherish her until death do you part?

Then please repeat after me: "I, Richard, take you, Gloria, to be my wedded wife. To have and to hold from this day forward. For better or for worse. For richer or for poorer. In sickness and in health. To love and cherish forever."

Gloria, in taking Richard to be your lawfully wedded husband, do you promise to love, honor, and cherish him until death do you part?

Then please repeat after me: "I, Gloria, take you, Richard, to be my wedded husband. To have and to hold from this day forward. For better or for worse. For richer or for poorer. In sickness and in health. To love and cherish forever."

At this time you will exchange the rings.

Richard, while placing the ring on Gloria's hand, please repeat after me: "With this ring I thee wed, and pledge my faith and loyalty to you."

Gloria, while placing the ring on Richard's hand, please repeat after me: *"With this ring I thee wed, and pledge my faith and loyalty to you."*

[Here I read "Sentry Dove"]

I would like to now share with you a Native American wedding blessing.

Now you will feel no rain, for each of you will shelter the other. Now you will feel no cold, for each of you will give warmth to the other. There is no loneliness ahead for either of you. You are still two separate bodies, but you will now walk this earth together. And may your days on this earth be long and good.

With the power invested in me by the state of California, I am honored to pronounce you man and wife. You may now kiss your wife.

3/20 Monday. Day 20

Thank You, with Love

Dear Tammy and Robin,

I really do not know where to begin to say thank for all you have done for me and for Richard these past few days. I am more than overwhelmed. My heart is full with love and appreciation. I am so very proud of both of you. I could never have asked for better daughters, ever.

The way you were able to organize a wedding in such a short time was unbelievable. You have done many incredible things for me over the years, but this really went above and beyond. The location was lovely; so much better than having the wedding at the house. I could look up at the mountains I love so much, see beauty in the world around me, and, as the lake flattened out, find some peace. Thank you with all my heart.

Thank you for the flowers, which meant so much to me. Any bride wants to be special, and that is exactly how you made me feel. With everything being done in such a hurry I was so surprised to see the bouquet. It was perfect. I couldn't have picked out a better one if I had done it myself. The freesias have a special meaning for me. I associate them with the first time Richard and I were together on the Isle of Man. Thank you for that special touch. All the way home to the Bay Area, I kept them by my side as a reminder of the beauty and effort you put into the wedding and how much you both must really love me.

Thank you for making all the arrangements, from organizing the food, finding the location, getting someone to marry us (who wasn't too religious), having a fire in the fireplace, and even having my granddaughter, Mylie, as a flower girl. She was precious. Thank you for doing that and for making all the phone calls and choices for me.

My mind has just been so numb. There is so much information I have to take in each day, and most of it isn't good. It is hard to cope and make so many decisions, and I knew planning a wedding was not one of them. The best news I received was when I got the phone call early in the morning and heard "Congratulations, Mom, you are getting married today. Don't worry. Robin and I will take care of everything." I couldn't believe it. I wanted to marry Richard so badly and wasn't sure it would really happen. I want to protect him and keep him safe. Thank you, thank you, thank you for making it a reality.

With tears of happiness in my eyes and love in my heart, I thank you again for everything.

I love you both very much.

3/21 Tuesday. Day 21

Dick is about to enter an unknown abyss today. It is deep, distant, and dark. There is no light and no sure landing. This abyss is filled with suffering and pain, both physical and emotional. It is the most difficult decision he has ever had to face. We know our family and friends are around the outside, ready to help in any way they can, but they can't—not right now. He has to do this himself, to make the decision that this path is the only one that may bring a good result. He is afraid. I can see it in his eyes. Today he will start to jump in—and I will go with him.

Today we visit the radiation center where Dick will have his radiation treatments. It is a lot better than I imagined. Even Dick thinks the people there are very supportive and caring. I never thought I would be in this world, but now I am. The doctor examines Dick and explains everything that will be happening during the next seven or eight weeks of treatment. Neither of us thought it would be that long. Originally we were told five to six weeks, and that amount of time would be hard enough. Dick is informed he cannot stop in the middle of the treatments, or his chances of success will be even worse. I had heard that over and over and now this—seven or eight weeks straight. How can a body withstand being cooked alive from the inside for so long? The doctor next describes the side effects of the treatments. He explains that Dick might lose his teeth; wind up with dry mouth and bad sunburn; be unable to eat; lose his ability to taste for many months, if not forever; and suffer a host of other terrible side effects. He takes a photograph of Dick for identification, because sometimes a patient's physical features can change so drastically. Once again I am numb but try to hold it together for Dick. I constantly remind myself to be strong. I must be his sentry dove at all times.

I ask questions, gather a wealth of information (more than I wanted to know), and generally try to keep informed. Dick is wonderful. He seems to accept what is happening to him and just wants to get it over with. He is still resistant to having a feeding tube inserted, but he will find out more about it when we see the gastroenterologist tomorrow. It will be another bad day. When do the good days come?

On the bright side, beautiful daffodils were being given out at the radiation center, and I took some home. They were supposed to be a symbol of spring and hope. I will look at them and try to believe.

The Unknown Abyss

Dick is about to enter an unknown abyss.
It is deep, distant, and dark.
It is filled with suffering and pain,
both physical and emotional.
There is no light and no sure landing.
Family and friends wait outside, ready to help.
There is nothing they can do.
This is his decision, his journey.
He is afraid and unsure but
today he will jump in . . .
and I
will go
with him.

3/22 Wednesday. Day 22

It is another difficult day. I should have known; it is a Wednesday. I hate Wednesdays.

We go to see the gastroenterology (GI) doctor to find out about the operation to have a PEG tube (feeding tube) inserted into Dick's stomach. The doctor explains that the feeding tube will allow him to get the nourishment he needs if he is unable to swallow well a few weeks from now. At that point, hopefully, he will not lose too much weight during the chemotherapy and radiation treatments, which would put him at even greater risk.

I ask the doctor what percentage of patients have the procedure done. I like asking doctors percent questions. It puts them on the line and they have to give a truthful answer. They don't like to, but they do. We are told that 85 percent to almost all patients have it done. Then the doctor describes the procedure itself. I can already see denial and refusal in Dick's face. A date for the operation is scheduled for the following month. Dick says in a soft voice as we leave, "I'll see." I can already tell this is going to be a struggle to get him to agree. All in all, it's been another hard day. Will they ever get easier?

On the bright side, we do not have to deal with doctors or hospitals until next week.

3/23 Thursday. Day 23

Today we are going back up to Lake Tahoe. I don't know why. I have already figured out that Dick will not be skiing, but we are going anyway.

Dick is a man who always likes to have the power—to be in control and be in command of his world and the world around him. He is the type of person to whom you can give any challenge and he will somehow figure out a good result. He is a successful engineer—the bigger the challenge, the better the solution. It may take him a while to find the best way to do something, but he always comes through. Whether it is building a million-dollar plant in a foreign country or a small conveyor belt to make something more efficient, he always has the answer. He is very creative and intelligent. I can give him any problem and he will solve it for me. I just take it for granted that he can resolve any crisis I might have. He is my pillar of strength and my protector.

But now he is not in control. I think that is why we are going back to the mountains. He is still trying to be master of something that has gotten the better of him, at least for the moment. He cannot find an easy solution as he does with all his other projects. He cannot write it out on paper and see the answer. He cannot control the medical system and the heap of paperwork he has to go through to even get started with his treatments. He has a type of frustration I have never seen in him before. He is angry with the cancer and with himself for not being able to solve this problem easily. So he is escaping—as if it will all go away—back to the Sierras and a few days of skiing.

On the bright side, the winter scenery is so beautiful. The royal-blue sky and marshmallow mountains are such a refreshing change from the city. Even I feel that it is an escape.

3/24 Friday. Day 24

Outside it is another lovely day, a perfect one for skiing or for anything else one might want to do. Inside it is a different story. I am right; Dick doesn't want to ski. I run a few errands and really accomplish nothing. He sits by the window and watches the birds outside. He likes doing that. I wonder what he is thinking. Dick does not share his feelings well; in fact, he does not share them at all. He also does not show emotion. I know it must be hard for him to see it is such a beautiful day to be out and for him to feel so different, so not like himself. Is he angry? Mad? Scared? Does he feel like screaming? Is he aware of how much his life is changing? How much he will no longer be in control? I can't tell. I wish I could know what is really going on inside him, but I decide now is not the time to try to open him up. I leave him alone. I'm dealing with my own thoughts and how I want to be out in the fresh air, free and happy, and not think about all these terrible feelings. I don't want to think about how much my life is changing too. Now I feel like screaming.

I build a fire at night and we sit close and watched television. We are in our own private world and, at least for now, nothing can touch us. We are safe and warm and together.

On the bright side, I love that we have a real fireplace. There is something about the warmth and beauty of the flames that always makes me feel happy and peaceful. That is what I need now, most of all: some peace.

3/25 Saturday. Day 25

There is a dark cloud over the house today, heavy, mean, and ugly. Outside it is snowing lightly, but inside it is very dark. Dick isn't feeling well at all. He doesn't want to do anything, and he is very tired. He lies on the couch and half-sleeps. I can't seem to get him interested in moving around.

I have never seen him this way. He is always doing something. I stay close by his side. He hasn't even started chemotherapy or radiation yet, and already he isn't feeling well. This is not a good sign. I don't know what to do; I feel so helpless. It begins to snow heavily, like the heaviness in my heart.

I finally ask him if he wants to leave the mountain and go back down to a lower elevation and home where he might be more comfortable and, in my mind, near his hospital. He says, "Yes, maybe we should." That is frightening in itself. Dick never admits anything is wrong or that he cannot have his way. I am scared now and my heart gets heavy again. I call for the road conditions. The road is closed because of the latest storm and downed power lines. We will have to wait until tomorrow. I now realize this will probably be the last time we are up in the mountains. I say a little prayer to keep him safe until the road reopens and we can get back to Bay Area.

At night, I stay close by Dick's side, trying to be of some comfort to him. I wonder if I am.

On the bright side, I was able to get the house ready to close up and will at least know all will be safe while we are gone.

3/26 Sunday. Day 26

The latest storm has finally passed, and I wake up to another beautiful landscape. It is one of those rare days with clear, deep blue skies and cold temperatures. It makes for a perfect powder day. In my heart I know we will not be going out to ski. I let Dick sleep.

We are going back down off the mountain. Dick hasn't felt well all weekend. This disease is beginning to rear its ugly head. I have never seen him like this. He never has a headache. He never sleeps during the day. He is always active. This is a different person. Something has gotten into him and I know what it is—cancer—and I am terrified.

The drive home is filled with unfamiliar feelings and concerns. I am glad we are back in the warmer climate. Later I go for a short walk and watch the cows in the field nearby. They have such a simple, peaceful life. They show little emotion and just graze as though they don't have a care in the world. Why can't our life be that way now?

On the bright side, I am glad I can feel emotion. Unlike the cows, I can feel the tremendous love I have for Dick. I am very lucky to have him.

I Am Terrified

You may not be afraid, but I am. I am terrified.
I am watching you get sick before my eyes.
Each day, each hour I see something in you
I have never seen before,
weakness.
You have always been my strength,
my pillar of steel, my rock and foundation.
You have always been there whenever I start to fall.
You are all that and more.
This cannot be happening, but it is.
I do not know how to stop it.
I have finally found something I cannot do.
I cannot fix this.
I am more than afraid.
I am terrified.

3/27 Monday. Day 27

I don't want to get my hopes up, but finally I am. While watching television this morning (something I never do this early, much less on that particular channel), I see a segment about a doctor in Pennsylvania who is doing a new procedure for cancer. At first I don't get too excited because there are so many different types of cancer. Then I hear "throat cancer" and see a patient who is being treated with a new state-of-the-art procedure. It allows the use of smaller instruments, therefore a less invasive procedure. The scarring and disfigurement are less, the need for additional surgery is less, and the recovery time is shorter. I can't believe what I'm hearing. Could this be something for which Dick could be a "candidate"? (Doctors love to use the word *candidate,* as though someone would actually run for the position of being sick.)

I glue my eyes to the set while I grab some paper and get the name of the doctor doing the procedure and the hospital where it is being done. I can't wait for Dick to come home to tell him. I'm almost afraid to get his hopes up, but I know this is something I can't pursue alone as he is the patient (candidate).

I sit Dick down and tell him all about what I've seen. He gets on the computer and tries to find the TV segment but can't. He then searches the hospital where the doctor is working and gets an e-mail address. Dick sends off a message explaining he has throat cancer and . . . then we wait. We wait to see if this busy, important doctor will even acknowledge his e-mail, wait for any kind of contact, even disappointment. We wait and wait, but not for long. Two hours later the doctor calls Dick in person! I can't believe it! My hopes go through the ceiling. Can this really be an answer for us? Is there really someone watching from above and our prayers been answered? Is this a sign? What???

They speak for a few minutes and the doctor asks Dick to

send his PET scan (a more detailed scan to look at the cancer) and CAT scan (X-ray that looks at the body in cross section) to him. I can't believe it. At least it is hope. Of course, we are running out of time. We have to go to the chemotherapy class tomorrow, and then Dick will probably be scheduled for chemo treatments. We also see the radiation doctor the next day and he will probably have his radiation treatments set up. There is so little time, but we will do our best. All I need is hope and I can do anything.

On the bright side, I have hope and Dick is finally getting involved with his condition.

3/28 Tuesday. Day 28

How many ways can someone get exhausted, drained, and numb all at the same time? I find out many of those ways today. We go to chemotherapy class. It takes all afternoon. The purpose of the class is to learn the ins and outs, good and bad of chemo—the process, the side effects, the places to look for help, and a ton of other general information, all very good, all very draining. It is after 5:00 P.M. before we get home, and neither one of us wants to eat. We are both numb. The brain can only process so much information at one time. I have had enough for today; maybe later, after I walk away from this for a while. Maybe then I will be able to handle it better—just not right now. Now I can't feel anything. I am exhausted and tired in a way I never knew possible. Not physically, but mentally, very tired. My brain actually hurts. There is so much to process. There is so much on the line. There is so much to do. Where do I start?

I have put my life on hold. I have canceled all my future plans. I closed up the house in the mountains and all that goes with it. I canceled all plans for us down here. Vacations, trips, dinners out with friends, weekends of freedom—all have disappeared. Now my calendar is filled with doctor dates, chemo dates, and radiation dates. My trips now will be to the pharmacy, hospital, support groups, and other cancer-related journeys. It is now time to take things one day at a time. One baby step each day, so my brain can comprehend all that is going on. I need to go slowly, so I am able to handle everything without hurting the way I am now, and I don't get too exhausted and fall apart. We both have a long road ahead. We must stay on the path; we cannot stray. Too much depends on it. No, *everything* depends on it.

In chemo class we are told how important the support person or caregiver is to the cancer patient and how much responsibility

73

is put on his or her shoulders. It is a heavy burden to carry. The caregiver needs strong shoulders all the time. I will be there. I will be strong, but right now I am still numb and need to rest. Tomorrow is another day.

On the bright side, it was good to know there are people in this world who do care about your well-being and are ready to help in any way they can, and to remember that I love Dick very much and will always be there for him, even if I am tired.

3/29 Wednesday. Day 29

Today is Wednesday again. How I seem to hate Wednesdays, especially this one. We had to go to radiation to have a mask molded to Dick's face. The idea is that they can use it each time he comes in to mark precisely where the radiation will be targeted. The hope is that then as little damage as possible will be done to the rest of his face. After that we had to go back to the hospital for Dick to get the PET scan.

The day turns into a total disaster. Dick has terrible claustrophobia. I always knew he had it, but I didn't know how bad it could get. At radiation he fights everything from the beginning. He is angry and mad no one will listen to him. He gags on the trays they put in his mouth. He goes crazy when they try to restrain him to keep his shoulders lowered in the right position while molding the mask. He hates lying on his back and has a horrible time breathing and starts to hyperventilate. Nothing works. They try to let him hold the straps himself so he can let go if he needs to and attempt to mold the mask again. Finally, they give up. Dick is a very difficult patient. They decide to call the doctor to give Dick a prescription for anxiety. A new date is set for Friday. Everyone is very understanding, except for Dick. He is already agitated and we haven't even gotten to the hospital for the PET scan. Also, he hasn't had anything to eat because of the PET scan and he is very hungry.

At the hospital Dick is no better. In fact, he is even worse. Now hungry and upset, he is already arguing he can't do it. We get the prescription filled and I give him the anxiety pill. Dick has never been one to take any medicine, so I think surely this will help calm him down. It doesn't. He reiterates that he has claustrophobia. I give him another pill. I tell him to try anyway. I say this is so very important and we have to send the results to the doctor in Pennsylvania. He says he will try. It is even worse.

Now he has barium or whatever they put in him but cannot do the scan. He describes how small the space is and that he just can't be put inside the machine. It is a disaster. Also Dick is agitated because he can't get his copayment back for the test. I think he is more upset by this than anything else. Maybe it is that this is the only part of his life he can control. He loses anyway; he can't get his money back.

On the way home Dick doesn't speak to me. He is more than angry—with the hospital, with the world, with me. All the way home I am crying. I'm crying because I feel that this was the last hope Dick had for the Pennsylvania doctor to review his case and, maybe, accept Dick as his patient. I'm crying because Dick gave everyone such a hard time and I was embarrassed, and I'm crying because Dick says he is so angry with me, he wants me to go away because he doesn't need me. I cry and cry and cry.

At home the pills finally take effect and Dick falls asleep on the couch. I go to bed and cry some more. I really hate Wednesdays.

On the bright side? Today, I could not find a bright side. I tried, but I could not.

76

3/30 Thursday. Day 30

Today doesn't start out well. We are both exhausted from yesterday. Dick gets the copy of the CAT scan ready to mail to the Pennsylvania doctor. I tell him, after all the trouble I went through to get the CAT scan released, the doctor really needs the PET scan too. Dick is still angry with me, and I am still hurt by him. Right or wrong, that is the way we feel at this moment. Dick leaves and says he will be at Has Beans, the one place where he feels safe.

I am still crying. I've only cried like this two other times in my life. One was when my mother died, and the other was at the end of my divorce, when I didn't know how I would survive. Now I'm crying the same way, a loud, violent, desperate cry I can't control. Maybe I need to hear it out loud; maybe I need to release everything that is still inside me; maybe it is just a normal part of the cancer process. Whatever it is, I'm crying for the third time in my life with real desperation.

Finally I stop. I realize I need help. I call every cancer support number I can find. There is a lot of information about groups but no one I can talk to at the moment. I don't want to call my daughters. They have their own lives and are very busy during the day, and I don't want to upset them. My other friends are at work. I am still devastated about how Dick is rejecting me. I need to talk to someone about his behavior.

I call a longtime friend who knew him even before I did. Bob is great. We talk and he finally calms me down. He tells me he knows how tough it is on me and Dick didn't mean all the things he said to me. He explains how important the caregiver is and that I need to take care of myself too. He says, "Hang in there," and he tells me to call him whenever I need to talk. I thank him for listening and say good-bye.

Dick comes back, and we talk. He had calmed down as well.

Anger had given way to understanding and realization that we are in this together. He explains his terrible fear of being enclosed but says he will really try to finish having the radiation mask made tomorrow. He says, "I know I have to do it or I will die." There—he has finally admitted the words to himself as well as me. It is a big turning point. We hold each other close, and the rest of the day gets better.

On the bright side, Dick loves me and still wants me around. Also, thank you, Bob, for being there today.

I Need Some Peace

Don't say, "Hang in there," when you don't understand what it means.

Don't send me twenty pounds of cake when Dick is nauseated and can't eat.

Don't invite me to dinner when Dick can't go out.

Don't say, "When he is feeling better, we will get together." I need help now.

Don't call early in the morning because it's the only time you have before work.

Don't call late at night when you get home, just to check in. We're already in bed.

I need some peace.

Don't send me flowers that will die in a week. Send me a plant that will live.

Don't offer to take me out. Bring me in a meal you cooked instead.

Don't leave a long message on the machine. Make it short and to the point.

Don't give me fifty different books to read about cancer. I am living with it.

Don't send me twelve hours of tapes on cancer. I need to get away from it.

Don't tell me I will be okay because I am strong. I am falling apart.

I need some peace.

Don't tell me you know how I feel unless you are dealing with cancer yourself.

I am in this deep, dark abyss with no way out, and cancer surrounds me.

Every day I smell it, feel it, touch it, hear it, and sense it.
There is little I can do.
I am barely coping as it is, and

                  I

                      need

                          some

                              peace.

3/31 Friday Day 31

Today is to be the big day. Either Dick is able to tolerate the
mask being molded on his face or there is no hope of him having
a chance to live. There is no other option and Dick knows it. The
time for Dick to be a patient of the doctor in Pennsylvania has
run out. It is now or never.

The radiation center calls and wants to move up his appointment time. I call Dick back from Has Beans, and although he
isn't happy, he comes right home. I give him one anxiety pill to
help him relax (yesterday I had given him two and it did nothing) and off we go to radiation. Not a great way to start but at
least he is going.

At radiation everyone understands about Dick's claustrophobia and they are ready for him. They try to do it as quickly as
possible. I can't stay in the room because of the radiation, but I
am allowed to watch him on the monitor. He doesn't move and
finally it is over. He does great! I can't believe it. My heart was
in my throat the whole time. I am floating high. Maybe this will
work out after all. Everyone else is pleased too, because they can
see there is hope for this difficult patient.

I ask if we can see the actual machine in the radiation room
where Dick will have his treatments so he can be more prepared.
In the room the technicians are very nice and explain what will
happen during the radiation procedure. Dick seems to understand and accept it. We are both drained but relieved as we
leave.

The rest of the day is mellow. Dick sets up a dental appointment for next week. We are told to take some precautions which
might increase his chances of saving his teeth. Also, five large
cartons of special drinks he had ordered have arrived. They all
need to be frozen, and I don't know where I'm going to find
room for them. He will need them when his throat is very sore

16

and becomes difficult to swallow well. At least it is good to see Dick finally taking an interest in his own care and beginning to look forward, which in turn is helping me. At least some of the burden is being lifted.

On the bright side, one big hurdle has been jumped. It is a very good day. We are both ready to fight this cancer all the way.

April

April

4/1 Saturday. Day 32

It is 4:30 in the morning and I cannot sleep. Dick is restless too. He tries to comfort me and holds me close. He finally falls asleep, and I slip out of bed to go into the other room to write. It is the only thing that saves me. I cannot call anyone at this hour. It is too early to go walking. I can't even scream, so I write. Writing down my thoughts is a release for me. It lets me feel what I am going through, lets me understand I have not lost my mind. It is my way of dealing with all that is in my life right now. Maybe someday others will read this too and understand.

I remember today is April Fool's Day. I used to like this day. I loved to play jokes on my friends. Maybe this nightmare I am going through is all a big joke, just a dream. Maybe I will wake up and laugh. How I wish it were true. To be able to make this cancer cloud go away so we could be the way we were, happy together, with no real worries. But the joke is on me, this is for real, I am not dreaming. It is going to be a long day and I am already tired. I join Dick back in bed.

We finally get up and have breakfast around noon. It is the latest we have ever stayed in bed. Already we can tell how much our lives are changing. Dick asks me what I want to do as we are never home on the weekends. We have always been out and enjoying life to the fullest on the weekends, whether it is skiing, motorcycling, sailing, or some other sport we enjoy together. Years ago when we first knew each other, Dick said, "There are fifty-two weekends in a year, and I want to spend them all with you." It has been that way ever since. Mother's Day is about the only exception. How do I tell him nothing is important to me now other than spending every moment with him, not only the weekends? I tell him to do whatever he wants as long as we are together.

The rest of the day is spent going to the grocery store and getting coffee at Has Beans, things we never do on the weekend. Dick is already aware of how much his life is changing, and he is not happy about it. He does not say anything, but I can tell. Also, for the first time in years, no one called and tried to play a joke on me. I think they know we have already been played the ultimate joke of all.

On the bright side, the mourning doves from last year have now moved into the planter full-time. We are naming the female Dovie. Maybe they are ready to have a family. Also, I went for a short walk nearby and saw the first of the wildflowers. That is good for my soul.

4/2 Sunday. Day 33

As usual it is raining outside; it has been all month. In fact, March went down as the wettest month in history in the Bay Area. It looks like there is no letup in April. Maybe it is like the tears I cry—endlessly. I try to do it when Dick is not around, but I still cry—a lot. I cry because I am frightened for Dick and scared for myself. I cry to let out all the pent-up emotions inside me. I get it out and then I go forward and function for the day.

This day again began with Dick getting up late. Maybe it is because he is up so much at night with trips to the bathroom; maybe it is something more. I worry. Another late breakfast now becomes lunch. He is angry with himself for feeling this way. We sit and talk about what is happening. He is worried he is spoiling my day and tells me to do what I want. I reply that I am, that what I want to do is to be here for him. I mention maybe we should start to contact some friends and get out. Maybe it would help him to talk to others about what is going on in our lives. He agrees. We call his oldest friends. They knew Dick many years before I came into his life. I know they will be very supportive. I am right. We agree to meet halfway between us; even though they live over an hour away, it's pouring outside and there will be tons of traffic.

It is the best medicine ever. We have a nice dinner together, laugh and talk about what is really happening. Dick does open up about his cancer and discusses the problems with hospitals and such. It is so good to see him at least acknowledge what is going on. Our friends even have a wedding card and gift for us. They are thrilled we finally got married. They know we are really good together. Dick explains he had for years called me a WIT (wife in training), and he had nearly given up. He says it was hopeless training me, and he might as well marry me. He tells them he now calls me his HM (house mouse) but adds FC

89

(first class). Everyone laughs. It is so good to see Dick as his old self with some of the tension gone. We part ways with smiles on our faces. We needed that.

―――――――――――――

On the bright side, friends are still the best medicine. Bob and Marilyn, thank you for joining us for dinner and for being our friends.

4/3 Monday. Day 34

Today is another day of Dick sleeping in. This new pattern of sleeping is beginning to worry me. I was warned he would be napping a lot when he was on radiation and chemotherapy, but he hasn't even started treatments. I worry, and then my stomach feels terrible. I do not need any excessive stress on me now. I have to get this under control, but I am just not sure how.

Dick finally gets up and we eat breakfast. I am trying to get him to not skip meals because he is already losing weight. He needs as much fat on him as possible so he will not get under-nourished while on treatments. I try but he is not very hungry, and we have to go off to see his dentist.

The dentist is great. He seems to understand the correlation between radiation and damage to one's teeth. He makes a mold of Dick's mouth so he can wear a tray filled with medicine to protect his teeth from bacteria. Too bad there isn't a tray he can wear to protect him from cancer, too. The dentist gives him several aids to help him, writes out instructions, and gives him a prescription for DentaPlus 5000, to help prevent cavities and strengthen tooth enamel, which Dick had heard about. Dick will come back again Wednesday for a final fitting of the mold. The dentist even comes out and talks to me about all Dick will be doing. I like him and feel better. Maybe this Wednesday will not be one I hate.

We finish the day with a trip to Has Beans and his usual latte. He seems to feel so safe there. I get my favorite iced drink with lots of whipped cream. I think it is good for both of us.

On the bright side, Dick is trying to do all he can to get ready for treatments, and that is helpful. All in all, we had a pretty good day.

4/4 Tuesday. Day 35

Dick gets up a little earlier today and showers. I think his feeling bad is over. I'm wrong. He still feels awful. On top of that he has a rash on his upper body I am worried about. He goes back to bed. I let him sleep and spend the morning writing and being quiet. It is still difficult for me to get used to this person with whom I am now living. Everything is so new. It is also hard because I am getting nothing done around the house or outside.

Dick finally gets up but only because the serviceman from Sears is coming in the afternoon to look at the washing machine, which is leaking. I tell Dick I can take care of it, but he gets up anyway. In the end, he just sits on the couch while I handle it. I can see he is a different person. It frightens me and I don't know what to do about it.

I do not know what to do about so many things. Dick's rash on his upper back is getting worse. I have heard one can get a rash from stress, and maybe that is what it is. Regardless, I don't know what to do for him. I tell him to call the doctor, but which one—his general doctor, the chemotherapy doctor, the radiation doctor, or the dermatologist? There are so many people involved, and in a big organization like Kaiser, it seems you just become a number. Even getting someone to call you back is difficult. It is very frustrating. Dick ignores my suggestion anyway.

Overall, it has been a rainy, depressing day and nothing much has happened. At least the washer got fixed so I can do laundry. Why isn't there a serviceman who can fix cancer and make it go away?

On the bright side, I now have clean clothes . . . big deal.

4/5 Wednesday. Day 36

Dick had to get up earlier today because he had to go back to the dentist. The molds would be ready. The dentist is excellent. He knows everything about the effects of radiation on teeth. He is even flying to Phoenix to give a lecture on the subject this evening. It is such a ray of hope, at least for saving his teeth. The dentist had even done research the night before, written down everything, and explained all the different routines Dick was to follow. He also gave Dick several different products to take home.

The trip to the dentist is good, but the next trip will not be. I have to deal with Dick and his taxes. He is mad because he has to get them filed before he becomes really sick. I say it must be done and set up a meeting for tomorrow. As usual, I am the one who has to take care of it, and I will do all the talking with his accountant. I am not very happy. Now I have to do all of last year's business and personal filing for Dick and get all the rest of the information we will have to take with us tomorrow. He doesn't want to deal with it; but then, he never has. It's a lot of work. I'm already tired and stressed. This is not going to make it any better.

On the bright side, as we came home there was a male turkey across the street and he was making some strange sounds, like a mating call. I answered back and he kept calling and looking around. We called back and forth to each other. It was great. The turkey even fanned out his feathers for me twice! That was a treat. I had never seen one do that in the wild before. Dick said we were both turkeys! At least he has not lost his sense of humor!

4/6 Thursday. Day 37

A lot has been going on today. Dick is still not feeling any better, and it is beginning to be a pattern. Again today he did not get up to go to Has Beans. He is not sleeping or eating well. This morning he just couldn't function.

We were supposed to see the accountant at 10:30 A.M., but I had to call and change the appointment to later in the afternoon. Then the condo I had put up for sale a few weeks earlier receives an offer. I need to make a decision right away whether to accept it. Although I don't want to take the offer, I agree and decide not to look back. My world has to be totally concentrated on Dick. I will not be able to cope with anything else. There are a lot of phone calls and paperwork back and forth, but at least it will be one more thing off my mind. This will also help me out financially. That burden alone has been a lot of stress.

Now we have to deal with the taxes. Dick is not feeling well during the whole trip to the accountant and I have to drive back home. A sure way to tell he is sick is when he doesn't drive. He does not relinquish command of the car easily. At least the taxes are done and I have one less problem to think about. I try to tell Dick we have to eliminate some of the extra stress and clutter in our lives so we can deal with this cancer head-on. We both need to be focused. I think he understands. It is not making his rash any better, though. He still will not call the dermatologist.

To relieve some of my stress I call my daughters. We talk about their pregnancies, sonograms, and general health. It is good to talk to them. It makes me feel a little area of my life is normal and safe.

On the bright side, today was the only day, in many weeks, it did not rain. It made headlines on the news, right after they talked about all the flooding, mudslides, and road closures! The real news, for me, is that Dovie, as we named the female mourning dove, is sitting on her nest full-time. It is wonderful to see her back.

4/7 Friday. Day 38

I write most of the morning while Dick sleeps in. Since he feels better when he finally gets up, he leaves to do some banking. I'm concerned because he is gone for such a long time. It turns out he was getting money transferred into a long-term certificate of deposit. I don't like that he has tied up funds for so long—what if we need it during his cancer treatments? I tell him so, but then I have to remind myself I should not care. Dick is just trying to protect me in case anything happens to him. I immediately let the issue drop. Then the phone rings.

We receive news our Tahoe neighbor has been killed skiing. It really surprises us both. Our friend was a very good skier and knew the trails well. We are told the visibility was not very good and he was going too fast. Also, he was not wearing a helmet. It is especially sad since he was very healthy otherwise and had so much to live for. Dick takes it especially hard, and the thought of mortality comes to the forefront in his mind. I try to comfort him. "See these arms? They are for wrapping around you," I say. "Don't get drippy," he answers. So much for comforting him.

Nothing much happens the rest of the day. We finally go to the store to get something for dinner. It is hard to shop these days because he doesn't want to eat much of anything. The irony of it all is that I love to cook. My cookbook collection numbers nearly a thousand. Actually, there are a lot of ironies these days.

On the bright side, if it can be called a bright side, between a fatal automobile accident we saw yesterday and the loss of our neighbor, we are both very conscious that death can come at any moment and not just from sickness. It has made us even more aware of how precious our time is together and how lucky we are to have each other right now.

I Have Him Now

Do not tell me of statistics that are not good numbers I know
the odds
but I have him now.

Do not let me worry about what if, what could have been, or
what should be:
I have him now.

Do not let me think bad thoughts but only good ones
because I have him now.

Do not say to me I have to accept what will be;
I have him now.

Do not talk to me in months or days or hours;
I have him now.

Do not let me believe anything but what I already do

because I have him now and now
is
all
that
matters.

4/8 Saturday. Day 39

We both slept late today, which is usual for Dick but rare for me. The reason was that Dovie somehow got spooked last night and flew out of her nest. She couldn't find her way back in the dark and was making a racket banging into the other plants and the window. I got up and turned the light on for her, but it did not help. She had a bump and blood on her head. I worried all night. It may seem silly with all that is going on in my life, but the doves give me a sense of pleasure and calm when I see them each morning. I enjoy watching them take turns caring for their eggs and love seeing the new babies hatch and grow. Even though they eventually fly away, I look forward to their coming back each spring. Dick enjoys them too, so I know he was concerned last night. Dick nicknames her Bumbles for the day. I am glad to see his humor.

While Dick sleeps on and off, I spend my time getting our paperwork under control—condo papers, tax papers, and other things that needed catching up. It is tiring and boring but I can do it without disturbing Dick, and at least I make some progress around here. I find this cancer is a two-man job—one to actually go through the process and the other to hold everything else together. I am that "other man."

Dick finally pulls himself together enough to go over to his sailboat, which is his pride and joy, and check it out after all the rain we have had lately. The car battery is dead so instead he has to get a new one and install it. He seems to feel a little better this afternoon. That is a good sign.

Later my girlfriend comes over and picks me up. We go to her office to design a wedding announcement. She is wonderful and does everything. At least I have a few moments to acknowledge we are even married! It gives me such a lift. I am also able to talk out some of my feelings and show her some of what I am writing. She says she will read it. It is also the first time I have left Dick since he found out he had throat cancer. I worry most of the time. It will also probably be the last time I will be able to leave him.

On the bright side, Dovie was back on the nest this morning and both doves did their morning swap. All is well in some parts of the world. Also, thanks for caring, Chris.

4/9 Sunday. Day 40

Today is our last day of freedom, the last day before we start spending every day with doctors, labs, hospitals, radiation rooms, and all the other places we do not want to visit. Everything we have been pushing out of our minds these past few days will come back with full force. Monday will be lab work, Tuesday will be the chemotherapy doctor and then off to another place for radiation X-rays, and finally Wednesday it all begins with a full day of chemotherapy and radiation treatments. I really hate Wednesdays. From then on our lives will never be the same. Of course, our lives already are not the same.

But for now we have a last day of freedom. For me it will be a day on which no one can hurt Dick and cause him pain, and a day we do not have to absorb more than we can handle. Today is Sunday and we have it all to ourselves. Dick is still sleeping while I write.

Funny how you think if you really have just one day to do something special, how hard it is to decide what to do. And as it turns out, there is nothing to decide for us. Dick is not feeling well most of the day; but we finally choose to go over to the boat and pump the bilge—not really exciting, but necessary.

We stop and get ice cream along the way to help his stomach. Hanging around a store is something we never do on the weekend. It feels so strange. I'd thought being on the boat would make Dick happy, but I think I was wrong. All he sees is that the boat needs work and he is probably thinking he might not be able to go sailing for a long time. I don't not ask him, but by the look on his face, I know. It is beginning to rain again so we come home. At least we spent the time together.

My girlfriend and her son stop over with a sample of our wedding announcements. She did a wonderful job and I am so thankful. I feed them dinner and they leave shortly after because

Dick is not feeling well. Maybe I should say "still," as he is never feeling well these days. I am worried because chemotherapy and radiation hasn't even started. Also, he is not eating right. I feel so hopeless. The abyss is getting deeper and deeper.

On the bright side, the announcements have my favorite wedding picture of the two of us.

I just want us to stay like that forever.

4/10 Monday. Day 41

Today we are going to the hospital so Dick can have his blood work done. Apparently it is drawn once in the beginning, again halfway through the treatments, and then at the end. I will be really stressed by the time the other blood tests are done; so much will be riding on them. For now, it is just an inconvenience for Dick. I think I'm going with him more to calm him down than anything else. A hospital is never a place anyone wants to spend time. When you are the patient and know you are going to be there a lot, it is even worse. Hospitals are for sick people, and it is just an in-your-face reminder that Dick is sick.

Since Dick didn't get up until late, the hospital trip is in the middle of the day. The good thing is that on the way back we stop by Has Beans. It's not quite the same, since the group of friends he usually sees in the morning is gone. I think he is beginning to realize how much his life is changing. It just doesn't seem fair—you work your whole life so you can relax in later years, and then something like this happens. Shit.

On the bright side, the sun was out at least part of the day today, before it started pouring.

4/11 Tuesday. Day 42

Today Dick has a hard time getting up. He doesn't feel well, is very tired, and his stomach is bad. Also, the gout he had years ago is beginning to rear its ugly head or, I should say, foot. On top of that, the rash on his back is worse. He has been losing weight because he hasn't been eating much, which is also not helping him. He is very edgy with me.

I know he doesn't want to go to the hospital to see the chemotherapy doctor. Apparently it is the usual routine the day before chemo. Yesterday's blood results are in and they do not look good. His potassium level is much too low and that is part of the reason he feels so tired and drained. There is a problem with his kidneys not functioning correctly, and his body is not taking in enough fluids. Although he drinks plenty of liquids, it doesn't seem to help. The doctor recommends that he drink Gatorade or Pedialyte to fight dehydration. Again, he strongly suggests having a feeding tube inserted into his stomach to help him through the next few months. We ask about X-rays for his stomach, have his rash looked at, and ask if it is too late to have a PET scan done. The answer is that nothing seems as important as getting him immediately into the "infusion room" to get an IV to rehydrate him and add potassium. He needs to be in better condition for the "big day" tomorrow. Also, one of the side effects of Cisplatin (the chemo drug he will be getting) is kidney damage. I never realized kidneys are so important and that you can die from kidney failure. Actually, I never realized much of what is happening to Dick. I was never one to go to a doctor, as I have always been healthy. This is a whole new world to me and a major wake-up call to become aware of my own health.

"Infusion" is an experience all its own. It brings reality right to the forefront. This is not a place for the meek, just the very weak. Two large rooms are lined with recliners and filled with very sick patients. It is very scary, very quiet, and very somber. We are told that once I accompany Dick in there, I will not be able to return if I leave. I decide that if Dick has to be there all day, I will be too. Also, only one person can accompany the patient and they are very strict—the doors are locked. This is not a happy visiting room with balloons and flowers. In fact, you can't even wear perfume or bring in strong-smelling food because the patients are so sensitive. The nurses are terrific, very patient and understanding, and are well aware of the gravity of the situation, both for the patients and for their caregivers. It is still a difficult time. Seeing Dick so weak and hooked up to an IV is brutal. I feel so helpless, and no matter how much of a sentry dove I want to be, there is so little I can do. I just sit by and wait, hour after hour. Finally, Dick feels a little better. He will have to return tomorrow and have his blood drawn again to see if he is improving.

Finally, it is on to radiation and another serious time. He has X-rays (they call them "films") and also another picture of him so they will know what he looks like in case his features begin to change too much (and to be sure they have the right patient). All in all, it is a hard day.

On the bright side, Dick was able to smile at me and forgot about this morning.

4/12 Wednesday. Day 43

Today is the day we start falling into the deep abyss. It is Wednesday. Whenever I hear the word, I know it will not be a good day. Today is no exception. Dick has to start his first chemotherapy and radiation treatments. It begins early, at 7:00 A.M., because there will be a lot of traffic on the way to the hospital. This is bad enough, but neither one of us really slept last night and we are already tired. Dick gets up a lot, which in turn wakes me up—that is, if I am sleeping at all. Also, it is pouring outside, maybe even harder than yesterday. Dick is feeling terrible and can hardly function. He is weak, looks pale, and does not want to eat; not a good way to begin. Later we have to go on to the radiation center for the beginning of his radiation treatments. It is going to be a grueling day.

Once at the hospital, Dick immediately has his blood drawn and is started on another IV of hydration fluids while waiting for the lab results to come in. They want to check his kidneys again, *STAT.* The results are not good. They are even worse than yesterday. His potassium level is really low and his kidney level is too high. A second IV full of fluids is started. At one point there are five different IV bags hanging from his stand waiting to pour into him—hydration solutions, nausea medications, and finally the chemo itself. We are there for more than five hours. It is very tiring, but at least Dick is able to be in a comfortable chair. He is so weak he doesn't even fuss when the needles poke into him. Eventually, he begins to feel better. The nurses are great too, which makes everything easier. Dick becomes more comfortable and relaxed. He finally falls asleep for a half hour, which gives his body a chance to rest. Five hours later, with a list of instructions and medications to take home, we are sent out again in the pouring rain to move on to the radiation center.

At radiation, even though we have to wait, all goes smoothly.

Dick is going to be a good patient. He has accepted that this is where he will be each day for many weeks and just wants to get through it. That is going to make it easier on everyone involved, especially me. On the way home, in the pouring rain and traffic, Dick is still telling me how to drive. Now I know he is feeling better.

All in all, it's an exhausting day, but at least we get through it. The doctors and chemo nurses are still worried about Dick's lab results. We have to go back tomorrow so he can get another IV full of hydration fluids. At least he is in the system and will be monitored closely. Best of all, we will have people to talk to if something starts to go wrong.

Back home I am more than tired, but I cannot rest. I have to cook dinner, unload the dishes, do the laundry, go food shopping, finish Dick's taxes, and make all the phone calls I didn't have a chance to do earlier today. Forget about doing anything for myself or coping with my own problems. Also, I will have to monitor Dick to see what reactions he has from the chemo and if he is going to be sick. Maybe I can just make dinner and let the rest go for tomorrow—after all, tomorrow is another day.

On the bright side, today is finally over.

4/13 Thursday. Day 44

One more tiring day begins. We are back to the hospital early so Dick can have another IV bag of hydration and potassium. The bag said "ASAP" on it, which is not a good sign. I was hoping his kidneys would be in better shape today, because we both need a rest. He is still not feeling well, and something is very wrong. More blood is drawn to see if he has to come back tomorrow. They have a hard time using his right arm. It is difficult starting so early doing something that is so unpleasant. He is given potassium pills by another doctor but told not to take them until someone calls. As usual, no one does.

Everything between the hospital and radiation is a blur. I think that is because I am so very tired. I tell Dick I need two hours to myself today while he runs errands. I desperately need to take care of me, get a good shower, do my hair, and otherwise feel like a woman again. I have lost feeling feminine these past few weeks. The sun is finally out and I just want to lie down for a half hour or so and soak up some rays. Dick calls it "playing lizard." I really need it badly. I am more than exhausted and just have no time to myself. Dick calls from the bank to tell me he is going to Has Beans and ask me if I want to join him. I really don't but I will drop anything if he wants me near. There went my two hours, but I did manage to get about forty minutes.

Then we are off to radiation at 5:00 P.M. in rush-hour traffic, but all goes okay. There is just no time to do anything. I can't seem to get caught up. I know I have to slow down or I will get sick, and then I won't be able to take care of Dick. It is just so hard; there is so much to do and no one else around to do it. I have taken to sticking little notes all over our kitchen cabinets so I won't forget all the things that need to be done—tons of phone calls and errands, as well as everything I have to do around the house (besides taking care of Dick). He really doesn't feel like doing anything these days. I certainly don't want to push him, so I do it all. There is just not enough of me to go around, and the weekend is coming up. I'm not sure what the procedure is for his care during that time. Everything is so up-side-down, and we will see a different doctor on Monday to have his potassium levels checked again as they are still very low.

Sadly, tonight we will not be able to go to a function that we had planned months ago, where we would have seen all our friends. It would have been good for both of us, but late this afternoon Dick is not up for it. I feel very sad and become even more aware of just how much our lives are changing. He takes Mylanta and it helps. He finally falls asleep on the couch.

On the bright side, the sun was out most of the day (which has been rare lately), a girlfriend left a lovely card for me personally at the door and, best of all, so far Dick has not gotten sick from the chemo.

4/14 Friday. Day 45

Dick has another IV this morning and his blood drawn again. How much more can they find that is wrong? Dick says everything "tastes like cat pee in your mouth," so he is not eating much. He does not take his nausea medicine because he says it makes him feel worse. I have my fingers crossed and am holding by breath.

I had called my daughters last night and told them it would be a last-minute decision whether to come down to celebrate both Easter and my birthday on Sunday. It is literally hour by hour to see if Dick will be up to it. His health will dictate. Also, they have to drive three hours in holiday traffic. Besides, it is just a day—we can always celebrate extra next year—hopefully. By afternoon Dick seems a little better, and so we decide the children might as well come down. I could use the help as well as the company.

On the way back from radiation, I see spring blossoms. It makes me aware we have left snow and winter just a short time ago and now realize we will still be here in summer. The seasons change. Will this cancer?

On the bright side, spring is a sign of freshness and new beginnings.

4/15 Saturday. Day 46

The really bright spot this weekend is that my daughters, their husbands, and my granddaughter come down. Dick is still weak, but we decided it would not only be good for my spirits but they could really take some of the burden off me. What a good decision. Dick and I spend most of the day at the hospital while he gets his IV of hydration and potassium, and so on. They all arrive mid-morning and immediately start working, even after the three-hour drive and with both daughters being pregnant.

They are terrific. They know just what has to be done (like, everything). They accomplish all the things and all errands I had been putting off. I had made lists for myself all over the house, and they find them and work as fast as they can to get as much done in the time they have. They know they will not be able to make any noise once we get back from the hospital, so they make every minute count.

When we arrive home, they are very respectful and quiet when Dick is nearby. Even my granddaughter is quiet because "Grandpa has a cold and is sleeping." Dinner is just leftovers from meals my girlfriends had previously brought over. We are all too exhausted to go out, and I don't want to leave Dick.

That evening my son-in-law teaches us to play rummy. For a few hours, while Dick sleeps, my children and I laugh and play cards and, at least for the time being, I am not drowning in the abyss.

On the bright side, laughter is good medicine for everyone.

How Do I Tell You?

"What do you want for your birthday?" Dick asks.
"For you to live, nothing more, nothing less," I reply.
How do I make you understand you are all I ever wanted in life?
When you came into my world, you made me complete and content.
You opened up not only new senses but new feelings as well.
I discovered emotions I never knew I had.
Passions I never thought I could experience.
I feel them deeply now.
I have a world of love inside me.
I want to spend the rest of my life sharing it with you.
You ask me what I want for my birthday.
How do I tell you all I want is for you to live?
I need nothing more.
I will accept nothing less.

4/16 Easter Sunday. Day 47 and My Birthday

Today is Sunday, Easter Sunday. It is also my birthday. To me, it is just another hard day. Dick is really sick and very weak. He had a terrible night and has been in bed since we got back from infusion yesterday at 12:30 P.M. It is hard to get him up because he is so sick and dizzy. We finally leave for the hospital to have an IV put in him again. Nothing is going right. His potassium level is too low, his kidneys are still not functioning correctly, he has terrible stomach problems from the chemo, and he is nauseated. He hasn't eaten since yesterday morning and says he can't take his medicine (which would help his stomach). It's a catch-22 situation and getting worse—and, of course, I am in the middle of it. Also, it is pouring outside; so much for a nice day, nice Easter, or nice birthday.

This is the first time in years I haven't skied on my birthday. I hardly have time to think about it, though. I am just in the "doing mode" today, no time for thinking or feeling sorry for myself. I am aware that this is the first time I have felt my age. I am sixty-three today and I feel every bit of it. Maybe I am just very tired.

On the bright side, my children are wonderful. While we were at the hospital my daughters and their husbands cleaned the house, including the refrigerator; changed the bed; cooked some food; did the laundry and whatever else they could think of to help me. They were like little heavenly angels for the day. I don't know what I would have done without them. There was not even enough time to thank them properly when we returned from the hospital. They had to drive three hours back to Lake Tahoe. With both my daughters being pregnant, I didn't want them tiring themselves out too much. So with a wave good-bye, and a kiss for my granddaughter, my angels were gone. Dick and I were alone once again.

Heavenly Angels

Thank you for today, for all you are doing.
I know it is more than I could ever imagine.
Thank you for taking some of the burden off my shoulders.
I need strong shoulders now for Richard.
Thank you for cleaning the house, running my errands,
and doing all I have not been able to accomplish.
Thank you for giving me that space of time so I can focus
on what I need to do—take care of Richard.
Thank you for being here in my time of need, to comfort me
and take away some of my fears.
Thank you for giving me the best birthday present of all.
On this Easter Sunday, thank you for being
my heavenly angels.
And, most of all, thank you for being my daughters.

—Love, Mom

4/17 Monday. Day 48

We have to go to radiation at 8:30 this morning in all the traffic. I hope there will be a better time slot soon, as this routine is exhausting. Dick's regular doctor is out so he sees another nice one. Dick is very weak and has not eaten for two full days, though he tried yesterday. Even my daughter's homemade soup doesn't stay down. He is not doing well at all. The doctor says it will get worse before it gets better since the radiation has not even affected him yet. He will feel the effects in about a week and a half from the beginning of his treatments. It is amazing how closely the medical profession has this all figured out, even though supposedly each patient is different. The doctor tells Dick he is scheduled for a total of thirty-five treatments and this is only his fourth, but that might change. He does mention that throat cancer in the back of the throat "is easier than in front on the tongue." I see this as a crumb of hope. He also mentions he has cured some—another crumb of hope.

Later, Dick sees a new male chemotherapy doctor who also is very nice. His regular female doctor is out sick. It is the best thing that could happen to Dick. I think he is willing to listen to a male doctor better—either this or Dick is so sick he is willing to listen to anyone. We discuss the fact that he is unable to take his medicines because he is so nauseated, he is not sleeping well, and he is getting weaker each day. The doctor prescribes suppositories to help with the nausea, orders more blood work since his potassium level is still down, and tells Dick to go directly to infusion for another IV session. He also prescribes more daily potassium IVs for the next week. The doctor again strongly advises Dick to have the PEG tube inserted now, as he is getting weaker and will wind up in the hospital. He needs the PEG tube appointment, currently scheduled for next week, to be moved up. The doctor says he will call over and see what can be done.

When the doctor asks Dick again if he is willing to have the operation to insert the PEG tube, Dick very softly replies, "I guess so. I have no other choice." The doctor asks Dick to repeat the answer clearly to ensure there is complete understanding on both sides. Dick replies, "Yes, I will have the operation." I hear it loud and clear!

On the bright side, I think Dick is finally becoming aware how seriously his life is threatened by this cancer.

4/18 Tuesday. Day 49

Our routine is a bit different today. We are up early to go to a hospital about a half hour away for his infusion. The idea is that the nurses there will be able to install a PICC line, a more permanent IV line that can stay in him longer. It will make it easier on Dick; he won't have to be continually poked every day to locate a new vein. The nurses were running out of places to find a good one.

After we get to the facility, Dick decides not to have the procedure done. I can't believe it! All the trouble everyone has taken to get him the appointment, and then to drive up there and he refuses it! Mad is not the word for what I am feeling. The infusion nurse knows I am upset and understands. I have tears in my eyes because I know it would make Dick's life so much easier and less painful. Also, I am mad because this is the third time Dick has come close and then canceled something important. There are too many very sick people who need all these appointments for Dick to be changing his mind at the last minute. Maybe it is his vanity, maybe he just doesn't want the tube hanging from his arm to remind him he is sick, or maybe he is just stubborn. The nurses see many male patients who try to hold on to control and have it their way. The nurse knows that in the end vanity goes out the window and winning any way one can is all that is important. Right now cancer still has the upper hand. We will have to change it.

Needless to say, this is not a good way to start the day. I am not happy. I guess the good thing is that he ate some yogurt this morning, 240 calories' worth, big deal. We'll see if it stays down. He hasn't eaten for three whole days, only sucked on ice chips. His potassium level is very bad at 2.5, the lowest it has been to date. If Dick does not start to respond he will end up in the hospital. The IVs dispense medicine but cannot give him nutrition.

He can't go on like this much longer.

No matter what happened earlier in the day, we still have to go to radiation at 5:00 P.M. in all the rush-hour traffic. I don't talk to him the whole way up and he knows I am still mad. On the way home he tries to rub my arm to let me know he still loves me. How can I be angry with someone who is so sick? I can't. After all, Dick is the patient and I have to go along with his decisions, no matter how I really feel. It is still painful and hard, but I love him so much and will stand by him throughout this whole journey.

————————————

On the bright side, we got through today and will be able to cope with tomorrow.

4/19 Wednesday. Day 50

Today we are back at the hospital in infusion for another IV at 12:30 P.M. The dietitian comes and talks to me. There is not much she can say, since Dick is not eating. Get the message? He isn't eating anything, so don't suggest any more soft foods or clever ways to get them into him. There, I think she finally understands—in any case, she goes away. At the same time, the social worker shows up. When we spoke by phone yesterday, I asked her not to come right at 12:30 P.M. but to wait until after Dick got settled. Here she is, all smiles with her little notebook, doing her job. I ask if she can come back later, because they have just started Dick on an IV and a nurse is taking his blood pressure and other vital signs. She gives me some information and asks if I want to go somewhere else and talk. I agree just to get her away from Dick, who is in no mood to hold a conversation with anyone.

The social worker gets an earful. I really vent when she asks me how I am doing. I tell her I am doing the best I can. I point out I am Dick's sole caregiver and do almost everything myself: I'm the only driver, I don't have family nearby, nor do I have a church support group. Additionally, I can't expect my two pregnant daughters to drive three hours to come help me. (Besides, their doctor told them they should not travel to different elevations soon anyway.) I'm also responsible for my ninety-five-year-old aunt who lives in New York. On top of all of this, I am dealing with the sale of my condo and all the phone calls and decisions that go along with that process. I inform her I have developed hives and they are getting worse. Before she can give me the speech about stress, I enlighten her that I understand the cause, but at the moment there is little I can do to alleviate it. (Maybe getting away from her would be a start!)

I tell her cancer support groups don't help if they are too far away and meet at times that won't work. I have already tried all those avenues. I convey to her that when I need someone, it is in the middle of the night when I can't sleep and desperately need to talk out my feelings. She shakes her head in sympathy. Big help. I calm down and explain I have found a solution myself, writing a journal, which seems to help me. I show her the volumes I have already written. She is impressed and decides I am coping better than most of the caregivers she has seen.

The session with the social worker is draining. I finally tell her I have to get back to Dick. She says that we will talk again tomorrow. (I think, *Don't hold your breath.*)

The GI doctor calls in the evening and informs us he has scheduled the PEG operation for tomorrow, but will go through with it only if Dick's potassium level is up; otherwise it will be too dangerous. He says to have Dick take eight potassium pills tonight and more tomorrow before he comes to the hospital. Dick takes six and then can't handle any more. We have to be at the hospital at 7:30 A.M. for blood work to check his potassium level again. The operation will be at about 11:00 A.M. We will then go from the hospital to radiation, if possible. He also mentions that we need to get the health care directive (which details which life-saving procedures, if any, the doctors can use) in to Surgery Admitting. Finally the day is over.

On the bright side, Dick will be able to get the PEG tube in sooner and it will be easier on him. No, it will be easier on both of us.

4/20 Thursday. Day 51, PEG Day

We are both up at 6:45 A.M., and I try to get some potassium pills into Dick. He can't swallow and he forgot to use the suppository to help with nausea before going to the hospital. This is not a good way to start.

At the hospital he goes to the lab and has his blood drawn at 8:00 A.M., then to Administration at 8:15 A.M. and hands in the health care directive and power of attorney (good that we had it ready), continuing upstairs to Pre-op Holding. Again his vitals are taken. By this time it is 10:00 A.M. and Dick decides he won't undress until we see that the operation will be a go. We wait and wait. He is not well and is weak and nauseated. Dick will be given antibiotics in the IV because of the increased risk from his being so weak. The PEG nurse comes by to talk about care and feeding procedures with the tube and I ask her to first wait to see if it is going to be done.

My hives are itchy all around my neck and into my scalp and now are spreading to my back. They are getting worse. I know it is from stress, but I can't do anything about it at the moment. Also, the condo pressures are not helping and I have too many phone calls to return, errands to run, banking to do, and on and on, never mind Dick's paperwork and forget about my care, which does not exist at the moment.

Finally, the doctor calls Pre-op. The operation will be canceled because Dick's potassium level is not high enough and it would be too risky. We are both exhausted and still have to go to radiation. It is a very long, discouraging day.

On the bright side, at least Dick was willing to go through with the operation.

4/21 Friday. Day 52

We are late for the hospital and have to rush to get there by 9:30 A.M. for another IV of hydration. I drop Dick off while I park and he manages to get up the steps by himself. He didn't have much for breakfast, only toast and a potassium pill. My hives are worse. This is definitely not a good way to start the day. At least Dick finally allows the nurse to leave his IV in for tomorrow. That is a big acceptance for him.

That evening, Dick's temperature is 100.3 and I start to get nervous. With chemotherapy, 100.5 is a danger point, and we had been warned to go to the emergency room if his temperature reaches that level. My girlfriend comes over and talks with us while we wait to see if his fever will climb any higher. She offers to take over calling a few friends to update them. It really helps me because I am so overwhelmed. I have no time, and I am in no condition to cope with all of them. I tell her about the episode with the dietitian and social worker and we both laugh. It is good for me. She leaves and returns with my favorite wine, a bar of chocolate, and a lovely card. Thanks for being there, Chris.

Dick has a bad night. The good news is that his temperature doesn't go up any higher. The discouraging news is that his gout is really hurting and aching. I try everything to help—cool cloth on his head for fever, cool towel on his foot to bring down the temperature. We are up all night. He has to crawl to the bathroom, which is both very painful and very scary to watch. I finally get a chair with wheels and push him back and forth in it. It is still very difficult to do.

On the bright side, having a friend is a beautiful thing to have when you are alone and scared.

4/22 Saturday. Day 53

What an incredible morning. After being up most of the night with Dick because of his gout, I have my first shower in days. My hives are not happy; they are even in my hair. I am worried about being able to get him to the hospital for his IV this morning, considering that he was unable to walk last night.

Unbelievably, at 6:40 A.M. my girlfriend calls to let me know about the fancy thermometer she has bought and left outside our door this morning on her way to work. (I don't think she was impressed with the old mercury one I was using last night.) She also says there are two cups of hot chocolate waiting there for us and a card. She asks how Dick is doing and I tell her about the difficult time I had moving him to the bathroom last night. Then, just as I am wondering how I am going to be able to get him to the car, she calls back and informs me she was able to get a walker and she will bring it right over. I can't believe it!

The walker really saves us and makes getting to the car so much easier and safer. She is truly an angel today and a friend who is pure gold. When it counts most she is here without me asking in every possible way—for support, to run errands, to give aid, everything. There are really not enough words to say how appreciative I am. (Also no time to thank her right now, but she understands.) That is the most important thing about a friend—one who understands. I've always told her she has missed her calling and should have been a nurse.

At the hospital I get a wheelchair and take Dick to infusion. I ask about getting a wheelchair for home and mention that his foot is very bad. The nurse in infusion advises us to go down to emergency to get his foot checked out. She says it might be a blood clot which could travel to his brain and Dick could die! She emphasizes the point and Dick finally accepts the fact that this might be serious even though he is sure it is just his gout.

We go down to emergency at 1:00 P.M. and are told he might need an ultrasound to see what is going with his foot. At 3:00 P.M. we are finally in an examining room but still haven't been seen by a doctor. The whole process takes hours. We are both exhausted, but it was the best decision ever to check it out. It turns out that Dick has something called cellulitis, which has many of the same symptoms as gout but is more serious. It is an infection that can travel up to the heart. I could just picture us back home at night trying to cope with gout and winding up in a much more serious predicament. The emergency doctor is very nice, prescribes antibiotics for Dick, and we finally leave the hospital after 5:00 P.M. Thank God, we don't have to go on to radiation, which is only on weekdays. It has been such a long and stressful day, I don't know where either one of us would have found the strength.

On the bright side, I am so very aware of what a good friend is and so very lucky to have one. Thank you a million times over, Chris.

4/23 Sunday. Day 54

Finally we have a day of rest. Dick is still recovering from being in the emergency room yesterday. It was very draining. His leg is not as swollen today, and his foot is feeling much better. The antibiotics are working. Today is just a time to rest and regroup.

Later his son and grandson stop by before they make the three-hour drive back to Lake Tahoe. It is good for Dick to see them, but it also makes him very tired.

After they leave we sit on the couch and discuss all that has been happening to him. I ask, "Are you afraid?" and he replies, "Only of losing you." I move closer and kiss him and answer, "You will never do that." No more conversation is needed. It is a good day of rest.

On the bright side, with those few words today Dick and I both know that our relationship is solid and strong and full of love. Nothing more is needed.

Are you afraid?

Only of losing you.

You will never do that.

4/24 Monday. Day 55

At last, a day that is not hell. I can't believe it! Today is the first day we don't have to spend hours upon hours in hospitals or with doctors. We only have to go to radiation in the afternoon. What a relief. Dick is able to sleep in and isn't so exhausted. I get up and do a few things. Playing catch-up isn't easy when you are so far behind. But at least I am able to take a step forward.

I let all the calls go to the answering machine. I have a girl-friend play secretary and call some of my friends to give a status report and explain that I am just overwhelmed. I get rid of some of the guilt I've been feeling and take a nice shower. I've been told taking care of the caregiver is just as important as taking care of the patient. Now I see why. When I am exhausted, I am not only unable to take care of myself but I cannot take care of Dick. I have been focusing so much on him and putting myself last, and it caught up with me. I have a terrible case of hives, which gets worse each day; the headache I have acquired lately never seems to go away; and I am drained. Today at least is a step in the right direction. After doing my nails, I actually feel human again and decide I can face the world. This abyss may be dark, but I am going to be able to deal with it.

Dick seems better too. This is a big step. The antibiotics he had been given for the cellulitis are apparently working. His foot is healing and he is walking on his own again—gingerly, but on his own. I am so glad we went to the emergency room. We both feel better today. He is beginning to eat too, not much, but at least a little. I think between me hammering it into him that he has to get some nourishment while he can still swallow, and the people at radiation today (who point out that he has already lost ten pounds), he gets the message. He eats just a little cereal, applesauce, and some peaches, but it is definitely a good sign. He has been losing too much weight. For me it is more than a good sign, it is hope. Also, a friend of his calls and offers to take him to radiation once in a while to give me a break. It will be like having a "get out of jail free" card! And finally, my trusted girlfriend arrives on our doorstep tonight with a nice casserole for us to eat. She has become gold—no, she always has been, I am simply more aware of it now. Thanks, Chris.

On the bright side, even though it was gloomy outside, it was bright in here.

4/25 Tuesday. Day 56

Today starts early, as we have to be at the hospital for two different doctor appointments. Neither one of us slept much last night. When Dick gets up I wake also to see if he is okay. He is walking better, but his mood has not improved. Is he scared? Depressed? I still do not know. He is not sharing with me. The GI doctor calls at 8:00 A.M. to ask what has happened regarding the PEG operation. He says he won't be able to do the surgery for a few weeks even if he wanted to because he is so booked up. I say I'll call him back after we see both doctors.

After arriving at the hospital, it is down to the lab for more blood tests. Next we see his chemotherapy doctor. She is more helpful this time and has up-to-date information about Erbitux (Cetuximab), an alternative to the chemotherapy drug Cisplatin, which Dick is currently taking. Apparently, it has about the same recovery period but is less invasive for the body. If he makes the change he will have to go once a week for six weeks instead of the three times now scheduled. I ask about Dick's kidney complication and if there is something to address the issue, not just fixing it with IVs of hydration and potassium. She doesn't have an answer since his potassium level is up to 3.1 on the latest test. We also discuss the problem with his vomiting and the fact that the medicines seem to irritate more than they help. Dick is finally feeling better, but it took him ten days and not the four or five she had predicted. He is not eating and has lost too much weight. She says to watch for changes or weaknesses and to see her again next week.

Then we see the primary oncology doctor who is overseeing Dick's progress. He isn't much help. We rarely see him, and it is too early in Dick's treatments for him to offer much of an opinion, even if he would. This doctor is quite cold. I guess someone in his position has to be, but it doesn't make it any easier on the patient. I tell the doctor the PEG operation was canceled by the GI doctor, not Dick, because Dick's potassium level was too low and it was therefore too risky. I ask if it can be rescheduled.

The oncology doctor sprays Dick's left nostril with topical lidocaine to numb it, and threads a nasopharyngoscope through his nose into his throat to see what is happening. It is hard to watch. Dick has swelling around his larynx (voice box). The doctor simply says Dick's "breathing is restricted" and to call him if Dick gets to the point where he can't breathe. A tracheotomy would then be necessary. The doctor said it casually, yet it sounded so scary. Dick has only had fifteen treatments and is already experiencing problems. This doctor will see Dick again in six weeks when all the treatments are over. About six weeks to go . . . it sounds like a lifetime.

And finally, we are off to radiation. It is a long day and when we go home, the GI doctor calls and informs us the PEG operation is now on for tomorrow. He goes over the list of instructions and says to be there early for more blood tests. I know everyone is trying very hard to do the best they can for Dick. This will be his only opportunity for the PEG surgery, since it is the original time slot booked before the operation was moved up a week. It is now or never.

On the bright side, six weeks isn't forever, even if it seems like it right now.

4/26 Wednesday. Day 57, PEG Operation

We are both very nervous going to the hospital today. Dick is still in disbelief that he has to have the procedure at all, and I am just praying his potassium level is up enough so the GI doctor can operate. They advise us to be there early so another IV can be started before the operation. After admissions and Pre-op, an IV of hydration is hooked up at 10:40 A.M., an IV of antibiotics at 11:03 A.M., and finally the potassium at 11:54 A.M.! After all the trouble the doctor went to, asking us to be there early for more potassium, the nurses didn't get the message and now Dick is going into the operation with barely any more potassium than he had in him yesterday. Needless to say, I am a bit unnerved and mad. I finally watch him all hooked up with different IVs as he goes into surgery. It is terrible. The good news is that the operation is going forward. The bad news is that my hives are worse.

Waiting and waiting, and waiting some more. It is something I have learned to do very well these past months. While Dick is being operated on, I am taken to a room to be shown how to feed liquid through the new tube. He will be given cans of high-calorie nutritional drinks (Isosource) made especially for the feeding tube. I feel awkward and unsure but am told I will get the hang of it. Finally, Dick is out of surgery and I can see him. We are both so glad it is over. The doctor comes in and says everything went well and gives us a list of instructions to take home. Of course, first we still have to go on to radiation. Radiation is like the postman—nothing stops it, not even an operation.

At home, Dick's feeding tube has to be flushed with water for the first twenty-four hours. Also the bandage around the feeding tube needs to be changed daily. I am very nervous doing it at first. I try not to show it because he needs to feel comfortable with me. All I can think is—I hope it works.

On the bright side, the operation went well and Dick should get stronger. One big step . . .

Numbers

How I hate numbers. There are numbers for everything in my world now, nothing else. There are numbers for blood pressure, heart rate, weight, pulse, and temperature. Every day those numbers are monitored. All the medicines are measured in numbers of centimeters and milligrams. I need a number to get in line to pick up prescriptions. I have numbers I have written down, page after page, so I can keep them straight. Even feeding has become numbers: seven cans of nutrition inserted into a feeding tube four times a day—two cans for breakfast, two cans for lunch, two cans for dinner, and one can in the evening. And then there are the numbers that are percentages: 80 percent chance a medication will have a bad side effect, 50 percent chance a treatment will work, 30 percent chance of survival. And numbers for times: one day a week for blood tests, seven days a week for IVs, thirty-five days of radiation, six weeks of chemotherapy, six weeks to see a follow-up doctor, and then numbers by months after that. And time is in numbers: time to eat, time to take medicine, time to go to the doctor. And the most important number of all is the medical record number. You're not a name but a number. No one even looks up at you until you give them this number, as if it is your only right to live or to deserve to be present.

Everything is measured in numbers, nothing more. Everything else is forgotten. What ever happened to the fact that we are people? Where are names? I do not want to live in a world of numbers. I want to live in a world of names. I want to remember all the names of the flowers I have learned while hiking in the mountains. I want to remember the names of my grandchildren, not the number of their years. I want to remember the names of all the good and caring people who have helped us along the way, not the number of times. I want to remember the names of words, such as *strength* and *hope,* that help me cope with this cancer. And most of all, I want to remember what words mean. Names of words such as *sunshine* and *sunsets, morning dew* and *evening calm, laughter* and *smiles,* and *gentle winds* and *happiness.* These are words that are important to me, not numbers.

Do not talk to me anymore in numbers. I am a person with feelings and a life. I am not a number or a statistic or an experiment. I am real, and I can feel and care and hurt and love.

I am myself, 100 percent of the time, and that is the only number I ever want to know.

4/27 Thursday. Day 58

This is the first day I am not the designated driver. A friend from Has Beans, who had also gone through radiation treatments, calls and offers to take Dick there today. I think it's wonderful, not only because it will give me a break but also because it will give Dick a chance to interact with someone else besides me. I am also supposed to go to Lake Tahoe and tie up all the loose ends with the condo. At the last minute Dick decides he wants me here and is unsure about being left alone. Of course, I stay. The condo can wait.

On the bright side, it is nice to know there are others around who are willing to help. Thanks, Vern.

4/28 Friday. Day 59

Dick wakes up hurting more than he did yesterday. Maybe the effects of the operation are finally taking hold, I don't know. I do know he is still not in any condition for me to leave him. I do need to be in Lake Tahoe, but I feel so guilty about going. I wish there were two of me. I wish this a lot these days—either two of me or that I had a lot of money. I have never envied wealthy people before, but at this point it sure would be nice to have the money to hire a driver, a cook, a housekeeper, a gardener, a nurse, and especially a secretary to keep track of all the appointments, medicines, and schedules I have now. In the meantime, I will have to make the best of it with just one of me.

For today, I make sure I stay close to him and check to see his feeding tube is working properly and he is taking care of it. I clean the wound around the tube every day and am becoming something of a surgical nurse with the care I give him. I know he appreciates it, though he doesn't express it now. He is still taking in a little food orally, but this is about to end. It is too hard for him. He has already lost almost thirty pounds since last fall. I don't want him to lose any more. For now, he is simply flushing water through the tube.

We are once again off for our daily trip to radiation. We will see what tomorrow will bring. This feeding tube has to be a success. It just has to be. . . .

On the bright side, the week is over and Dick will have a weekend when he does not have to go to the hospital for an IV of hydration. It will be like a mini-vacation.

136

4/29 Saturday. Day 60

Today is a day of firsts. It is the first time Dick takes in nourishment through his feeding tube (one complete can) and it is the first time I am leaving Dick by himself for more than a few hours since all this chaos began. I make sure he is able to flush the tube on his own. This is a big step toward him being in charge of his own care.

I have to go back to Lake Tahoe overnight to close up the house properly and tie up loose ends, as we had left in a hurry the previous month. In addition, I have to turn in the final papers for the condo sale. It will be one less stress off my mind and body. Originally, Dick had planned to go with me, but he is not strong enough. I confirm that his son will still stop by and take him to see his boat, but after that Dick will be alone. I go by myself, but the guilt is terrible.

The three-hour drive up is good for me. My hives are finally beginning to go away. I think it is the fact that I get to see the mountains I love so much. Maybe it is also that, for a few hours, I can run away from the cancer and all the pain. It is still hard for me to let go. I worry so much about Dick. It is also the first time I have been alone and had any "down time," if I can call it that. I get everything done that I need to—finish the real estate transaction, pack up clothes, see one daughter, and close up the house. I call in the early evening to see how Dick is doing, and he says he is fine. I still worry.

The plan was that I would stay overnight and return in the morning. When I call Dick again later in the evening, he is not doing well and I want to come home. He doesn't want me driving the twisting mountain roads in the dark and says to come back in the morning. In the end, I should have gone right away. I don't sleep most of the night and when I leave, at seven the next morning, I am exhausted and drained. I will not leave him again unless he has someone else there to take care of him. The stress is just too much for both of us.

On the bright side, the mountains are still there and the fresh air felt good in my lungs.

4/30 Sunday. Day 61

I arrive back from Lake Tahoe early in the morning so I will be there when Dick gets up. I am exhausted from worrying about him all night and having very little sleep. Even though I accomplished a lot, it was a mistake to leave. Dick and I are joined at the hip now, and it will be no good when we are apart.

Also, this turns out to be a hard day. Cancer is showing its ugly self. Dick is feeling the blisters in his throat. It is sore and he is beginning to have a difficult time swallowing. I hurt so much for him. I tell him I wish I could share some of his pain. He replies that he would never want that for me. Also, it is a hard day because he is feeling weak. He isn't eating enough, and it is catching up with him. He is able to get two and a half cans of nutritional drinks in him, but it is not enough; the nutritionist wants him to have at least seven cans a day. He has lost weight and it is really beginning to show. His feeding-tube incision is sore, and this is bothering him. He is walking very slowly and acts like an old man. He walks as though he is in much pain. It is a side of him I have never seen — vulnerability. It is very difficult to watch. I know he is beginning to be scared and to realize this cancer is serious. He still has not opened up to me, no matter how much I ask. I do not try to press him, but I am so worried about his mental condition. I give him space, but it is not easy.

He is sleeping a lot today. Maybe it is good, at least for now, for him to be in peace. I continue to write and try to make sense of all that is happening to us. "Why" still creeps back into my mind, but I know there is no answer. It is just a useless thought. This is a hard day.

On the bright side, I went out into the yard and smelled the new apple blossoms. Spring has finally arrived, and it is a welcome sight.

Why

Sooner or later, the question had to come.
Why? Why Dick? Why us?
I know no amount of crying will answer the question,
but that is all I seem to do.
I know anger is a wasted emotion, but that is all I feel.
I know being sorry for us won't make any difference,
but that is what I am.
I know what *is* is, and shit happens, and that is all I know.
I just want to know why. I will deal with the rest.

May

May

5/1 Monday. Day 62

Today is a good day. Dick begins to take the nutritional drink willingly through his PEG tube. He even asks for it when he gets up! This is a big breakthrough. I know it is hard for him to accept what is happening to him. He is very stubborn and does not want to give in. However, he is finally beginning to admit he just may have to have help. Afterward he feels better, no stomach problems, no nausea! I tell him it is because he isn't starving his body anymore. What a blessing! At least the pressure of seeing Dick get weaker and weaker before my eyes is alleviated. Hopefully this will turn things around.

The bad news is that he only accepts the tube feeding because his throat is getting worse. He said he was beginning to feel it a little on Friday and a little more throughout the weekend. Now it is really beginning to hurt, just as his doctor predicted and right on time. It is amazing how the medical profession knows the routine so well they can predict a patient's reaction schedule quite accurately. Even though there are more than one hundred different types of cancer, each of which can affect patients differently, there are still many similarities. Doctors know much of what lies ahead, and yet everything is still so new to us. We don't dare predict anything, much less look to the future. We just remember, one day at a time . . .

Additionally, the bad news is that his cellulitis has come

back. He didn't take his antibiotics regularly, and now we have to deal with his foot again.

―――――――――――――

On the bright side, although I am still exhausted, I know it is temporary and I will eventually feel better.

5/2 Tuesday. Day 63

Sometimes you just know it is going to be a bad day. This is one of those times. Dick's foot is really hurting him and he has a fever. He can't walk well and has to use the walker to go to the hospital for his doctor's appointment.

Upon arriving, his potassium level is checked and is now under control so he does not need to take pills. At least one good thing has happened. Dick has changed his mind about the chemotherapy drug Cisplatin and is now going with Erbitux. It is an antibody that is not supposed to be as harsh on the body. It is designed to suppress the growth of the cancerous cells. He got so nauseated with his first treatment he did not want to go through it again. As he says, "The cure is worse than the disease." The chemo doctor acknowledges that the standard Cisplatin they used was rough on him and agrees that maybe, since he had such a difficult time, Erbitux is a better choice.

Doctors have their certain protocol and do not like to deviate from it. None of the other twelve doctors in the oncology department had ever prescribed it before. Although they had heard of it, no one had seen it used. Actually, I was the one who mentioned it to Dick, as I had read about it recently and about the clinical trials that had been done. I am still unsure of this drug because it had yet to be proved to work on throat cancer, and was previously used to treat only colon cancer. I feel that Cisplatin, no matter how tough, is the established choice. With his cancer being so advanced, I want him to have the best chance for success.

In the end, as always, it is the patient's decision, and all I can give is my opinion. Other times, I had been very certain, but this time I am not as confident. Nonetheless, I will stand by Dick's decision. It will not make him as nauseated and maybe he will be able to eat better. Instead of three treatments of chemo a week, he will go once a week for six weeks, with the first time being the longest to determine if he has any allergic reaction. The biggest side effect would be fatigue, and he might get a bad rash much like acne. The side effects can show up anytime during the course of treatment. However, he would not have to take all the chemo medicines. We will see.

In the meantime, he is able to take four cans of the nutritional drink through his PEG tube. He must work up to seven cans just to maintain his current weight and keep his strength. Every day seems to be a struggle, and today is certainly no exception. At least our daily trip to radiation goes smoothly.

———————————————

On the bright side, I saw Dovie's baby! Mother and baby are both doing fine.

5/3 Wednesday. Day 64

We have to be at the hospital early because it will be a long session. This is going to be the first time Dick is given Erbitux instead of Cisplatin. He will be in infusion until the afternoon to make sure there is no negative reaction. The hardest part of trying any experimental or new drug is the stress of deciding what works best and the fear of making a life-threatening mistake. I research everything I can find, yet I still feel like such a novice. Doctors and nurses can only do so much. The crucial decisions have to be the patient's alone. I still struggle with my own thoughts, but I will continue to stand by Dick's decision.

After chemo it is on to radiation, and finally we return home, still watching to see if there would be any negative side effects. Dick seems to tolerate this much better and does not get sick. My only concern is whether it will work. *That* is the million-dollar question. Maybe this will enable him to tolerate his nutritional drinks better. He is still not getting enough. I will have to try to get him to take more tomorrow. We are both just so tired, and it has been a very long day.

On the bright side, Dick has started down a different path knowing I will always be by his side, and that has made our bond even stronger.

5/4 Thursday. Day 65

Again today we wait to see if there will be a reaction to the Erbitux. We decide Dick is tolerating it well. He is quite pleased with his decision. He is even able to have more cans of nutrition, and this has pleased us both. Maybe it is the beginning of better times . . . or maybe this treatment will be a sleeping dog lying in wait, with disastrous results. We will not know for another month or so. One of the hardest things about cancer is the uncertainty—the not knowing, the guessing, the wondering, and especially the waiting . . . waiting for appointments, waiting for test results, waiting for drug reactions, and especially, waiting for miracles. Waiting and waiting. In the meantime, it hangs heavy on my heart, and I think about it every day. I do not know what Dick thinks about it, because he still will not share anything with me. I don't understand how he is able to hold so much inside him. Is it because he has always been a very private man, or does he not want to worry me?

On the bright side, it is good to see Dick not so weak and nauseated.

5/5 Friday. Day 66

Finally, this is a better day. Dick at last has all seven cans of nutritional drinks, three thousand calories, the amount he needs each day to sustain his weight. He cannot afford to lose any more because he has already lost so much. It is such a relief to see him maintain this amount and be comfortable. One more step in the right direction . . .

Also, this is a better day because not one, but two of my girl-friends stop by and leave all kinds of goodies for me. They are really the ones who are keeping me going, as I do not take care of myself and my eating habits are terrible. They bring food, treats, cards, and friendly smiles. They also keep my spirits up.

But best of all, my daughters and my granddaughter arrive in the evening to celebrate an early Mother's Day weekend with me. We had decided to spend this weekend together, instead putting them through of all the traffic and hassle involved with next Sunday. Since they are both pregnant, I know they would like to spend Mother's Day with their husbands, and I understand. However, for now, I need to spend time with my family, for comfort, and familiarity, and love. This is the best medicine for me, as well as the best Mother's Day present.

On the bright side, it was a good day, and I am looking forward to a great weekend. That is really something, as I usually have not let myself look forward to things at all.

5/6 Saturday. Day 67

We are all up early. It is a special day for my daughters, granddaughter, and me. We are going to spend the morning going to the more than forty garage sales our neighborhood holds on this weekend each year! We have been planning it for a few weeks. My daughters love going to them.

We have a delightful time. It is uplifting to be out of the house and not going to the hospital or anything heavy and depressing. Also, it is great to be with my children and laugh. Knowing Dick is taking it easy at home and able to get his nutrition into himself enables me to relax even more. We drive and drive, shop and shop, laugh and laugh. It is wonderful. Do we find any real treasures? Maybe not, but we have a treasure of a day. I love my children so much, and every minute I get to spend with them is precious. Moreover, having my granddaughter around, and buying her treasures at the garage sales, is even more fun.

Leaving Dick is still hard. Guilt is a big part of my life now. Why am I the healthy one? Why can't I do more to help him? How can I be so selfish as to leave him? Where do I separate my life from his? Do I deserve a separate life at all? In the end, knowing we are nearby and have cell phones makes it easier to reduce the guilt, if only for a little while. Even the best of caregivers needs some time apart from their ill loved ones. Space and time can be a good thing.

That evening I convince my daughters that we need to play rummy. Then we laugh some more. All in all, it is a good day.

On the bright side, it was a happy day and I won at rummy!

5/7 Sunday. Day 68

After the excitement yesterday, we all sleep late. I also want to spend more time with Dick as I still feel guilty about leaving him. He is happy for me and glad I can get out, laugh, and not worry about him all the time.

My daughters want to take me out for a special Mother's Day lunch. I tell them I don't need anything; their coming down has been special enough, and they shouldn't waste their money. Instead I suggest we pick up some sandwiches at a deli and take my granddaughter, Mylie, to the park. They think it's a great idea. What a few hours it was! We have a chance to sit in the sun and relax while Mylie runs around in the water fountains. She has a wonderful time, and it is so nice for me to enjoy the time with her. My daughters buy me special cookies to have with my sandwich. It is the best Mother's Day lunch ever. I know it is easier for all of us. With them both being pregnant and having to drive three hours back home, we just need some peaceful downtime.

Sometimes it is easy to forget cancer not only touches the cancer patient and caregiver but also the others who care and worry about them. Cancer has tentacles that manage to reach everywhere. My children are able to see that I am still able to hold things together, and they will now not worry as much about me.

Eventually it is time for them to leave and we say our goodbyes. It is hard, because I miss them very much. Back in the house I cuddle up to Dick and hold his hand. I have so much love inside me to give. I am a very lucky lady.

On the bright side, it doesn't take a lot of money to bring happiness. Sometimes the smallest and least expensive things are the best.

5/8 Monday. Day 69

As morning breaks today Dick starts to have a difficult time swallowing water. He begins choking when he tries. It gets worse all during the day. It sounds as though he is going to die every time he attempts to put anything down his throat. I knew it was just a matter of time before this would start, but I am not ready for it to happen so soon. I give up everything to stay near him as he struggles. I can't even write. When I see the look of fear and discouragement in his face, I begin lose hope and feel myself beginning to drop deeper into this abyss. Yesterday, up in spirits; today, so far down. When will he get a break? When will I?

––––––––––––––––––––

Where is my bright side now?

5/9 Tuesday. Day 70

Today Dick is unable to swallow water at all. Nothing will go down his throat, not even medicine. He is able to take in the seven cans of nutrition through the feeding tube. Thank God he accepted the operation for the feeding tube.

Why, why, *why* is all I can ask again. Why must Dick suffer so much? There is always something more that goes wrong to make things worse for him. Now he can't even enjoy eating. I hate to see him in so much pain and feel there is nothing I can do for him. I am getting so discouraged. . . . There comes a moment when we all reach our limit. Today I have reached mine...

———————————

I am not sure I can even find a bright side today . . . and tomorrow is another Wednesday.

Why

Sooner or later, the question had to come.
Why? Why Dick? Why us?
I know no amount of crying will answer the question,
but that is all I seem to do.
I know anger is a wasted emotion, but that is all I feel.
I know being sorry for us won't make any difference,
but that is what I am.
I know what *is* is, and shit happens, and that is all I know.
I just want to know why. I will deal with the rest.

5/10 Wednesday. Day 71

We see the chemotherapy doctor early today before Dick's treatment. We tell her he needs his stomach medicines in liquid form, as he can no longer swallow pills. In fact, he is not swallowing anything at all, not even water. This is especially hard for Dick since he was always one who actually enjoyed drinking water. Even when we would go out to dinner or be invited to someone's home, he would ask for water instead of wine or liquor.

She prescribes a liquid pain medicine and an antifungal medicine to help with the heavy saliva now building up in his mouth. The good news is that he has continued to take the full seven cans of liquid nutrition. Dick's weight is beginning to stabilize, and he is beginning to feel better. I also ask if it is okay that he sleeps a lot and the doctor says it is fine. An appointment is made for two weeks from now, again prior to his chemotherapy treatment. Additionally, he still needs blood work done each week the day before.

We are able to get into infusion early for his IV of Erbitux. This is helpful, as waiting is sometimes the hardest thing to do, and we are there for such a long time. Also, there is usually not a lot of time between his chemo and radiation treatments. We will now have to travel around with his cans of nutrition in case we can't get back home between trips. I do not want him to break his schedule of feedings now that he is getting comfortable with the feeding tube. I think the hardest part for Dick accepting the feeding tube is that he sees it hanging out of his body every day. It is a constant reminder that he is seriously ill. It makes him aware that he is not the invincible man he thought he was, that he is actually quite fragile. I see the look on his face when he has to clean out the tube and his annoyance with the whole process. It is one part of this journey on which I cannot help Dick, either

155

physically or mentally. The best I can do is to assure him my love is unending, no matter what he looks like or what his condition.

Then it is off to radiation and finally home. Overall, it is a very long, draining day. Wednesday; I hate Wednesdays.

On the bright side, Wednesday is over and tomorrow is a brand new day.

5/11 Thursday. Day 72

Dick is not feeling well today. A friend from Has Beans was supposed to chauffeur him to radiation so I could go to Lake Tahoe early, but Dick decides at the last minute that I should take him. I think the effects from the Erbitux yesterday are beginning to show. He is also starting to have a hard time speaking because his throat has become so sore from the radiation. Either way, I think he has begun to realize how very serious cancer is, and just maybe, he is aware that he will miss me. In any event, I put off going to Lake Tahoe until tonight.

The radiation doctor had told us Dick would really take a beating from all the radiation and warned us about the blisters that would form on the inside of his throat. The doctor said it casually, as he deals with this effect every day. We do not. Neither one of us had any idea what this really entailed. Dick has begun to speak less and less, and we are beginning to enter a silent world. It was hard enough to try to find out what he was thinking while he could speak, and now it is becoming impossible. I know he must be feeling shut out and like the world is closing in on him. I get him a whiteboard so he will be able to write down what he wants or needs. So far, he has left it blank.

My world is closing in on me as well. It was bad enough when I stopped cooking for Dick and we could not eat together, but now we are not even able to share in conversation. My world is getting darker and smaller. I must remember to keep the light in both my heart and my spirit.

For my spirit there is Dovie, who has returned to make a second nest in the deck planter. I can't believe it. It has been only four days since she left with the baby bird and she is already back. There is one big egg there, so I will not be able to move her now. Rats. Boy, is she a horny little devil. I don't know how we will both get through this round, since her nest is right outside the door this time and I need to water the other plants nearby. We will see—just what I need is another challenge.

I finally get somewhat caught up with the house, but I am paying for it by being so tired. I am not looking forward to driving up to Lake Tahoe tonight. I check to see how Dick is doing and tell him there will be no good time for me to leave and that he still has harder times ahead. He seems to accept it. I call a girlfriend to be on standby and finally leave around 7:00 P.M.

In the end, the drive up is not as bad as I had expected. There is a full moon out and the mountains, even in the dark, are beautiful. I feel like I'm coming home to a safe and happy place.

On the bright side, it is nice to have Dovie trust us and be able to see her baby when it is born, even though she causes us problems because we can't water the plants around her.

5/12 Friday. Day 73

At Lake Tahoe I have so much to do and so little time. There isn't a moment I don't worry about Dick and keep my cell phone nearby in case he calls. Even though Dick cannot really speak, I will recognize the number and can immediately start back. Caregivers have it so much better today with the invention of cell phones. It does give a certain amount of freedom and flexibility.

I put our ski equipment and winter clothes away. This is hard: the last time we used our skis, we were so happy. I wonder when the next time would come when we would be able to ski or, more important, be so happy. I rake up a few pine needles in front of the house so it looks as if someone lives here, check around for leaks or other problems, reset the timer, leave to run errands, and stop by to see one of my daughters. I am tired and don't feel well, so I stay there for an hour. I know it will make me late getting back, but Dick is covered. His friend, Vern, is taking him to radiation today so I can be in Lake Tahoe for these hours. Also, I think it will be good for Dick to have some male companionship instead of just me. Although he can't really speak now, I hope he can make an effort and try to express himself.

I finally feel a little better and drove home. The mountains are beautiful in the daytime and so refreshing to see. I needed to refresh my soul, too. I miss them so much and feel peace here. I wonder when I will ever find complete peace again. Back down in civilization, the traffic is terrible with a horrible accident, just another reminder that life is fragile and never to be taken for granted.

Once home it is so good to be back near Dick. I know I will have a hard time leaving him from now on. Moreover, I know he is glad to have me back—not that I can do anything, but just so I am around like a warm, fuzzy blanket.

On the bright side, some stress was lifted off my shoulders today, which helps a lot. It also helped seeing the beautiful, crisp, snow-laden mountains and reaffirming that this is still a beautiful world and we are all such a small part of it.

5/13 Saturday. Day 74

Dick sleeps most of the day. He is not doing well and had a difficult night. He couldn't sleep because his stomach gave him problems. He looks very tired and drained. I feel so helpless. There is only so much I can do, and then I just have to stand aside and watch Dick suffer. This is the hardest part, simply standing by. Like a ball game in which you know you could hit the home run but it is not your turn, so you just stand there and wait for the results. I just stand by and wait, but this is no game.

A girlfriend from San Francisco comes over for an early breakfast with me. It is good to see her and to get out. I need it. Dick knows I do, too. I spend so much time hovering over him that I do little for myself. It's important to interact with the real world. I live in such an isolated world now, isolated and silent. My girlfriend and I talk for hours, and at least I hear the sound of my own voice—the worries, the hopes, and the fears. I can feel and let it out. I tell her I am writing a journal and show her what I've done. She thinks it is a great idea and says I should publish it to help other caregivers understand the process and all the feelings and uncertainties that go with it. I agree; I wish I had known before all I know now. It would have made some of this easier—no less painful, but at least I would have been able to understand more.

The rest of the day I spend catching up on my writing. It feels good. I need some kind of release, and Dick is still not ready to talk, even if he could.

On the bright side, it was refreshing to be out in the world with other people and communicate. I also saw a deer on the hillside.

5/14 Sunday. Day 75

It is Mother's Day. What a mother of a day. I hardly slept at all last night and feel terrible today, partly from being tired and partly from being sad. I didn't sleep well because I tried to snuggle next to Dick in bed and every time I tried to touch him, anywhere, it hurt him and he was uncomfortable. I just needed to be cuddled and have the warmth of his touch, and he was unable to respond. I was hurt and sad and lonely. I cried. I got up and went into the other room to write. I wrote for hours and let all my feelings out. I cried for myself, for Dick, for all the bad things that happen in life to anyone. I just cried and cried, alone where no one could hear me. It felt good, and then it was over and I continued to write. Even some of my own prose overwhelmed me. And I cried again. Finally, hours later, when I did return to bed, Dick reached out and held my hand. It meant so much, and I finally slept because I knew I was not alone.

This is the first Mother's Day my children and I have not been together. I am overwhelmingly aware of the loss. I know they were here last weekend, but still, I am a mother and it hurts. Maybe I am just feeling sorry for myself. Maybe I am just very tired.

I spend a lazy day, the very first one I've had—no hospitals, doctor appointments to go to, nowhere we have to be. Dick sleeps most of the day, and I take it easy and write. I don't even get dressed or clean the house, not even the dishes. I need this to be a day of rest, my Mother's Day present to myself. I even "play lizard" in the sun for a few minutes and catch up on calls I need to return. I feel guilty, but it is necessary. I don't need flowers, candy, or even a fancy dinner. I need this.

Gloria Burola McSorley

On the bright side, I am very, very lucky to be a mother and have wonderful children, whether they are nearby or far away. I know we will always have a close bond. Thank you, Tammy and Robin. Also, thank you, Kathy, for bringing the salmon over for my dinner. It really made it seem like it was a special day.

5/15 Monday. Day 76

Dick had a terrible night. He coughed and coughed with the thick liquid that now forms in his mouth. It is as thick as corn syrup on a cold, dreary morning, and he gags on it, which in turn wakes him up. Because of the location of the radiation, the saliva glands are not functioning correctly. He even throws up around six this morning. He is very tired and not doing well at all. I can already tell this is going to be a tough day for him.

The condo sale is finally finished, and I pay off loans. Every bit off my plate will help in these coming months. While Dick rests this morning, I work on his medical records, bills, appointments, and so on, and get them filed and organized. There is so much to deal with each day. I keep a notebook with all the information we acquire and take it with us to every appointment. It has helped out many times. It is one small way I can help Dick, and I need to help him in every way I can—and it helps me, too. I had known these treatments were going to be hard on him, but I didn't understand how extremely exhausting and draining they would be on me as his caregiver. I thought I was very strong but I am feeling whipped. I never seem to get caught up and barely have time to take care of myself.

No time to think now, it is off to radiation, which turns out to be a disaster. Dick can't complete the treatment and starts to gag and suffocate. Afterward, we figure out it was the thick saliva in his throat that was causing him problems. We go to see the doctor, who suggests he constantly take the antifungal medicine he has and continually swish his mouth out with baking soda and water. He will try it tomorrow.

On the bright side, Dovie has two eggs in her nest, not one. Following her progress and watching her babies hatch is something I do for my own sanity.

5/16 Tuesday. Day 77

Dick continues to have terrible nights. Night after night seems to be the same. He was up until 3:00 A.M. and I was awake with him. He was coughing up the heavy saliva. Dick has been warned the saliva would get thick, but neither one of us thought it would actually choke him. The doctors never stress how impossible this is going to be. They just use the word *discomfort* and play down the real difficulty and problems with this stage of treatment. Nowhere and in no way did either of us anticipate this amount of torture. He eventually takes the antifungal medicine and seems to improve. As usual, it isn't until he is exhausted that he gives in to it. He seems to be doing a lot better this morning and even takes his medicines, including Salagen (for dry mouth), on his own. They seem to be working so far.

But we still live in a silent world. Dick is unable to speak with me or anyone else, even if he wanted to. I share this world as well. Not being able to talk and share my feeling with the one person who is my best friend, my partner, my love, because he is unable to respond is both frustrating and discouraging. The isolation of being alone, the quietness, and the loneliness are sometimes the hardest parts of this journey for me. Nevertheless, no time to dwell now; it is off to radiation.

At radiation he appears to have more color in his face, and he is even walking better. When I ask him to write down what he is feeling about all of this, he gives me the finger. Now I know he is doing better.

And finally, back to the hospital for blood work again. All in all, today has been Dick's best day in quite a while. He is more awake than he has been in about a week. He even tries to speak. He also seems to have a bit of a personality again. Maybe some of the fear is gone. His color is back and today I have more of a husband than a patient. I tell him he looks better too. I think that gives him hope. Even after radiation he stays awake for the evening, which helps him sleep better. He still has to get up a lot to go to the bathroom and clean his mouth of the heavy saliva, but all in all, I think it is his best day in a long time.

On the bright side, I am happy to have my husband back and new hope.

5/17 Wednesday. Day 78

Wednesday is chemotherapy again. This will be a hard day. We are greeted with an ice chest full of food from a girlfriend as we leave the house. Everyone is trying to be so helpful.

At the hospital we have a very nice nurse, and Dick feels comfortable with her. The nurses can make such a difference in a patient's care. They should be appreciated more. I sit and watch all they do each day, and I am in awe about where they find the strength to be so positive and helpful. I wonder how much of the patient's pain and suffering is translated into their own lives and how they handle the stress and the workload. They are the ones who are at the forefront of this disease, and the liaison between the doctors and the treatments. The doctors prescribe what needs to be done, but nurses see to more of the patients and follow up with compassion and care. I have gained a tremendous understanding and respect for all they are able to do and the strength they have shown.

It is still hard see Dick connected up to the IVs (three today), Erbitux (Cetuximab), sodium chloride, and Benadryl. At the same time, he has Tylenol put through his feeding tube as well as his two cans of nutrition. At last, he can rest. After that, it is twenty minutes back to the house for a quick salad for me, more medicines for Dick, and then off again forty minutes back for radiation.

Finally at home, I am too tired to see my girlfriend when she stops by to pick up her ice chest. Week after week, my exhaustion builds at the same time as Dick's strength wanes. Wednesday is always a hard day.

On the bright side, spring has finally arrived, it's beautiful outside, and I was so tired I actually liked my salad, which is not my favorite. Thanks, Kathy.

When Does Tired End?

How tired is tired? There seems to be no end.
Every day, every moment, every night,
I feel life ooze out of me as if I have been trying
To stay in the water too long
And I am drowning.

How tired is tired?
When I no longer have the energy to eat?
When going to the store is too much of an effort?
When housework no longer seems possible?
When taking a shower is more of a chore than a pleasure?

How tired is tired?
When my brain can no longer balance a checkbook,
Follow medicine instructions, or set appointment dates?
When I cannot hold a decent conversation?
When getting up to move hurts all over, inside and out?

I do not know.
But there is still much to do in the days ahead.
All I do know is that I cannot be tired now.
But
I
Can
Still
Ask . . .

When does tired end?

5/18 Thursday. Day 79

We are both so tired, and we had another bad night. Dick is feeling the effects of his chemo, and all the good that was happening to him yesterday is ebbing away. Damn, this seems so unfair. I am not getting anything done. The house is a mess, the yard has not been looked at in months, I have no energy, I look a mess, and I am discouraged and worried that the freight train we are on is picking up speed. At least for now we know, more or less, what to expect each day. At the end of his treatments, we will get the results and see what can be done. I do not even want to think that far ahead. For now, I am just in the coping mode. I take everything a little bit at a time. To do more is too overwhelming. It doesn't change anything, but taking baby steps makes the problems a little easier for me to deal with on a daily basis.

More and more, I live in this silent world. Dick still cannot speak at all. He is mostly sleeping. I do not eat with him because the smell of food bothers him and, I think, it is hard for him to see real food when all he can have are the cans of nutrition that go through his feeding tube. Without being able to enjoy and look forward to eating, his world has become so much harder. At night, I cannot be near him because of his feeding tube and because he is so uncomfortable and hot from the radiation. I am beginning to feel very lonely—that is, when I have a chance to feel at all. I'm sure Dick feels the same.

At radiation, his doctor says Dick's treatments have been changed a little (he does not say why) and he will have to continue until the end of the month. I had hoped radiation would be finished before the Memorial Day weekend, especially since that Sunday is the anniversary of the day we met so many years ago. I am too tired to figure out if it is more days of treatment than originally planned. Tomorrow I will think. Tonight, just let me sleep.

———————————————

On the bright side, my daughters called and they both had a 3-D scan and are doing well with their pregnancies. Tammy found out she is having a boy. I am very happy for her.

I Am Scared

I look at you while you are sleeping.
I see your hair has started to thin.
I see your face so tired and drawn.
I see your smile no longer exists.
I see your body has become weak and frail.
I hear your breathing shallow and labored.
I sense the pain you feel with every breath.
I smell the sickness that surrounds you.
I know you will not wake for hours.
I know I will be by your side.
I am scared, but I will not show it.
So begins another day.

5/19 Friday. Day 80

Dick and I did not sleep again and were up all night because of his saliva problem. I seem like a broken record to say this every day, but each morning when I get up I realize I had hoped the night before would have been different—better, easier, or both. It never seems to be the case. I am very tired and unable to function. Every day I seem to get further behind, accomplish less, and become more exhausted. I drive for us, think for us, cope for us, decide for us, and, of course, speak for us. We had always shared everything, every decision, every plan, every desire, and every moment. This has become an unbelievable life for me, one I could never have imagined and was not warned about. I had been told to rely on family and friends, to have faith, and to hang in there, but no one can walk in my shoes and help me cope with my exhaustion every night. I am alone, and I feel it in every way possible; and the silent world I continue to live in does not make it any easier.

Except for going to radiation, today has been peaceful and uneventful, other than that the rain has come back, which is quite an event in itself for this time of year in California.

On the bright side, I am glad the week is over and we can rest. More important, we can begin counting down his final treatments, with seven more to go.

172

Do You Know How Tired I Am?

I am your nurse to clean your wound, take your temperature,
and monitor your very being.
I am your legs to run your errands, be around when you call
me, and anticipate your every move.
I am your voice to communicate with doctors, explain your
pain, and express all you cannot.
I am your ears when you are too weak to hear or understand
what the doctors are saying.
I am your secretary to keep track of all your appointments
with doctors, radiation, and chemotherapy.
I am your memory of medicines that need to be taken and pre-
scriptions that need to be filled.
I am your driver to doctors, chemotherapy, radiation, the
pharmacy, and the million other places I need to go to take
care of you.
I am your schedule for when to eat, when to sleep, and when
to take your medicines.
I am your strength when you are too weak to stand, too tired
to cope, and too discouraged to go on.
I am all of this and more.
Do you know how tired I am? I do.
I am so tired today. Maybe tomorrow will be better.
But whatever tomorrow will bring, I will be there
to be all
that I am
for you.

5/20 Saturday. Day 81

Today is an easy one for me. Dick sleeps all day because he feels awful, very hot, and his throat is really hurting him. I catch up on my writing. It makes me feel better to get something accomplished and tie up loose ends. I write downstairs while he lies on the couch upstairs resting. I give him a bell to signal me if he needs anything. I am now like Pavlov's dog and obey quite well. I hope someday I can be untrained.

Finally, keeping the cell phone by my side, I run a few errands. Our friends are calling less now because they know Dick cannot speak. They don't want to disturb him, but mostly it's because they really don't know how to help. Our world is getting much smaller each day. At least with a cell phone I can get out and rejoin the real world. My life has changed drastically, being in this silent existence with Dick. I long to get out and communicate with "normal" people. It is still difficult getting used to being here on the weekends, because I am so accustomed to going to radiation every day. I forgot we didn't have to go today, and this allowed me time to get caught up.

———————————

On the bright side, Dick rang his bell and showed me a mother turkey and twelve babies outside our house. It was the best thing ever, because it was exciting seeing them close, and because Dick is aware how much I would enjoy them.

174

5/21 Sunday. Day 82

I have cabin fever. After another horrible night with no rest; we are both exhausted today. Dick makes up for the lack of sleep by napping most of the day while I work. I have to do everything for both of us. All the responsibility, all the decisions, and all the work are exhausting. Then there is the mental aspect of all this cancer—the worry, the watching, having to see his suffering, and the frustration of being able to do so little. I don't dare take a nap now or I will never sleep tonight, and I have a feeling it will be another bad one.

But I do have cabin fever. First, it is raining hard—unusual for this time of year. This eliminates going out in the sun to lift my spirits. Second, since Dick is sleeping most of the time, the house is quiet, and I don't even hear the sound of my own voice. I would love to be able to get out and scream. Instead, I clean the house, do the laundry, and catch up on a few things. More important, of course, I write, my saving grace.

I would still love to know what Dick is thinking and what he is really feeling about all he is going through. He still won't open up, and now I can't even get him to use the computer to express his thoughts. He is just too tired.

I spend the afternoon alone and watch a ball game, from start to finish, for the first time in my life. Definitely things have changed around here. Sometimes it feels as if I were living on another planet, an alien world, and I cannot find my way back to a familiar one.

On the bright side, I guess I am making progress around the house.

175

Who Am I?

Who am I? I do not remember. All I am called now is Mrs. So-and-So, the patient's wife. "Oh, your husband is not in? Can you take a message?" As if I'm not capable of being anyone. "Will this date be okay with him?" How about it being okay with me? Remember me? I am a person.

I think I still am, anyway. I used to be—before cancer, before I became just an extension of the patient, a necessary part of the team to keep him going. I am the part who runs his errands, helps him with his medicine, changes his dressings, prepares his special foods, drives him to the hospital, is there for hours on end, and helps with all the questions that need answering. "Yes, my husband is not allergic to this or that." "Yes, his birthday is this and his medical record number is that." "Yes, I will drive him home and take care of him."

Who am I, you ask! I am his wife, his loyal companion who is here every minute of every day, of every week, of every month, and now for this year and on and on. I am always here, even though I don't have a name, even though my thoughts and wishes have become nonexistent, and even though I have had to cancel my world for the past year. I do not remember when I last made a date to do something for myself. What self? I don't even know who I am. I am lost. I do not matter, and sometimes I don't even know my own name.

"How is your husband?" "Is he getting better?" "When can he come out and play?" How about me! When will someone ask how I am? When will someone ask if I am well? When will someone ask if I want to come out to play? Oh yes, you don't know who I am, so you cannot ask. The problem is that I don't know either.

Who am I?

5/22 Monday. Day 83

Dick is not feeling well. He sleeps most of the time before we have to go to radiation. Once there, I talk to Aleece, another cancer patient, who is scheduled each day about the same time as Dick. I show her what I have been writing. She says she loves it.

Dick is taking a long time, so we talk some more. We discuss what the caregiver goes through. It is good to have another perspective. Finally, Dick comes out. He could not put the tray in his lower mouth because it made him gag. That was why it took so long.

It is a bad sign. I already feel the fear and uncertainty of what this could mean. Dick needs to complete all his radiation treatments, not some but all, and without interruption. The technicians are wonderful and patient. They have a special, gentle way of dealing with and understanding the defenselessness of cancer patients. They tried everything they could think of today to make it possible for Dick to complete his radiation treatment, but with his claustrophobia taking hold, nothing seemed to work.

The doctor is called in and suggests that Dick bring the numbing medicine with him tomorrow. They will try to see if it makes the process any easier for him. Dick has to finish all his treatments. There is too much at stake, and there are only six treatments left. I give Aleece an orchid I had brought with me and we leave.

It is going to be a long, hard night of What if? What will be? What will happen? I am not looking forward to it.

———————————

On the bright side, thank you, Amanda and Hernando, for being so tolerant with Dick. Also, thank you, Aleece, for your thoughts; they are very helpful.

177

5/23 Tuesday. Day 84

Dick has another bad night, just like the nights before. How many times can I say that? Another bad night, like it is normal. Late at night, he begins to have labored breathing. The saliva builds up to such a point in his throat that he is choking. It is horrible to hear. It sounds as if he were dying.

Neither one of us can sleep. He gets up and goes to the bathroom, tries to get the saliva out, coughs a few more times again, and returns to bed . . . and then it starts all over again—the difficulty breathing, the gurgling sound in his throat, the struggle to get comfortable so he gets up, over and over and over. It goes on for hours. The medicine he has been given does not seem to work. I don't know what to do. I am exhausted, but I know he is worse.

I am discouraged and at a new low point in this journey. I am feeling desperate, and am having a hard time finding a bright side today. Of course, it is only 7:30 in the morning. I will have to give the day a chance. Dick has a chemotherapy doctor appointment today, and we will discuss the problem with her. Something must be done. He still has six more treatments to go, so he will be getting worse. Then it will be another two weeks before he will begin to feel better. Where will either one of us find the strength to last that long?

The chemotherapy doctor appointment goes okay. Dick is checked and all my questions are answered. I explain again how Dick struggles at night with breathing and choking on the saliva. She understands but only says to rinse with the medicine again (the one that doesn't really work). So much for help there.

Then it is off to radiation and a total disaster. Since Dick had such a difficult time yesterday, the radiologist has suggested he take some medicine right before the treatment that will numb his mouth. It doesn't work. It makes him worse and, more important, it makes him frightened. His throat closes up and he feels as though he were choking; worse, he feels claustrophobic. He has a horrible look in his eyes. It is imperative that radiation be completed every day—only on the weekends does it stop—and he must have all thirty-five treatments, the maximum amount. The body can't handle any more. The day has become a failure. Another day is added to his total treatment and we come home. I am devastated. I am not sure if Dick realizes how crucial this is, or if he really cares anymore. How much can one person stand?

———————

On the bright side, Dick is sleeping; at least for the moment, one of us is out of pain.

179

Where Do I Go to Find Strength?

Where do I go to find strength?
There must be a special place to go
when I am at the bottom of my helplessness.
Is there a place that is safe and secure,
a place to feel warm and restful?
Is it holding a young child's hand,
or in a grown daughter's arms?
Is there solace and strength in a church
or in family or friends?
I do not know where this place is.
It seems to be eluding me,
and I need to find it now.
I am tired and weak
and there is not enough of me to go around.
I need to be strong and steady and resilient.
So please tell me,
where do I go to find strength?

5/24 Wednesday. Day 85

Another long, draining day, one of extreme highs and lows. We had another night of no sleep, with Dick up coughing and choking because of the thick saliva. Today it is back to the hospital for his IV of Erbitux. Hours of sitting by his side while the fluid drips into him. I hate Wednesdays. Additionally, I think the infection around the feeding tube looks worse than it did yesterday, even though the doctor has said it was looking good and I was doing an excellent job. I clean it every day just as a surgical nurse would, and I am very careful.

Today I am on pins and needles because Dick could not do his radiation treatment yesterday and I know he has to do it today. It just might save his life. I ask him to please try for me, if not for himself. The tension on the way to radiation is terrible. I can see Dick is anxious, too. I ask him to be sure he can do it before we drive all the way up there (and I get my hopes up too much). He motions that he thinks he can. We decide he will rinse his mouth very well just before going in to have the treatment. That way the saliva might not be too thick and would not choke him. I have my heart in my throat the whole time.

He does it! What a relief. The emotion I feel is overwhelming. I did not know I had so much inside me. Driving all the way home, I silently cry with relief, tears rolling down my cheeks. Dick is too tired and drained to notice. I am glad.

At dinner by myself, I have wine and a brownie to celebrate. At radiation yesterday I had given Aleece an orchid to say goodbye. Today, she was just finishing up the last of her treatments and she brought me a brownie. It was so much appreciated, food for the soul as well as the body.

What a day it has been. I feel the best I have in a long time. While Dick rests, I write—volumes. It feels good. Finally, I feel better and have a peaceful end to the day.

On the bright side, it is good to be able to see some light, however dim it may be. It was also good to know there are really good and kind people in this world. Thank you, Aleece.

How Do I Thank You?

How do I thank you for making my day?
How do I tell you how much it means to me to have your gift?
A simple gesture, a simple brownie,
How can I tell you it means so much more?

The past few days have been more than hard,
More than anyone would want to experience.
Draining, exhausting, frightening and depressing,
Fearful for life itself.

Dick could not do his radiation treatment.
My world was coming to an end.
My life would be over without him,
And radiation was the only hope.

Time stopped, my heart stopped, living stopped.
But today he was able to finish his treatment.
It was the beginning of the end.
Only a few more to go.

I was finally able to relax.
All the way home, I cried.
With joy, with relief, with every emotion in me.
And at home I was ready to celebrate.

I ate and drank a favorite wine,
And with it I had your brownie,
So perfect, so welcome, so wanted.
How do I thank you for giving me hope?

5/25 Thursday. Day 86

Dick sleeps all morning after another night of wakefulness. I try to be quiet and work around him. Dick is as much of a zombie as I am. The constant up and down at night has left him in a fog, a tiring, depressing, useless fog, and I am right there with him. A night or two one can cope with loss of sleep, but after weeks this is becoming unbearable—and yet there are still more days to face.

Dick has now taken to writing on the whiteboard anything he wants to communicate to me, as his throat is so raw and painful. I live in a completely silent world. It was hard enough not being able to touch him, but it is especially hard not to hear the voice of someone you love. It is a loneliness that is difficult to explain.

This cancer is so unfair. Of course it is, I know. When cancer can attack a small child who has not had a chance to live or torment the last years of a person's life so there is no peace, it is not fair. The ups and downs cancer brings are not fair either. When hope is the one thing everyone needs to be strong and deal with all that is to come, cancer has a way of sneaking up and robbing you of it. It is so unjust, and so hard to fight this unseen enemy.

At radiation Dick struggles again. They have to stop his treatment and do it in two parts. The technician comes to me and asks what the problem is, and I again explain that the saliva is so thick in Dick's throat that he gags and chokes on it while he is lying down for his treatment. Since he can't breathe, he panics, because Dick has claustrophobia. They are very understanding. Everyone there is so nice and very patient. Dick is at least able to finish his treatment, and he is told he only has four more to go. We are finally counting down to the finish.

Gloria Burola McSorley

On the bright side, it is wonderful to know there are patient and sensitive people in this world willing to help. Thank you, again, Amanda and Hernando.

5/26 Friday. Day 87

Today is an easy day, if you can call it that, because Dick's radiation treatment is called off. The radiology department calls this morning and says the machine is broken and it will be down all day. I am worried he will miss too many days, what with Memorial Day coming up. They say it will not be a problem since he is so near the end of his treatments. It still does not give me a warm fuzzy feeling, but there is nothing I can do about it.

I catch up on a few things, go grocery shopping—the first time in forever—and work on my zillion plants. I know I should get rid of some of them now that I do not have any extra time, but they are like my babies. I love watching them grow. Of course, the one Dovie nests in is dying, but that is allowed. I make a mess; nevertheless it is good therapy for me. The house too is more than untidy, but I can clean it tomorrow. It will be a long weekend, and I will have a chance to get a step ahead. It is more important to have a glass of wine with a girlfriend who comes over after work. She even brings dinner, and we talk about all the good times we have shared over the years. This is cleansing to my soul, which is much more important than a clean house, any day.

On the bright side, I am very lucky to have friends who care about me.

5/27 Saturday. Day 88

Today is a quiet day; I know Dick will sleep most of the time. I have accepted this, but it is still hard to be so alone. Also, I can't make a lot of noise, so I don't get much done around the house. I do the best I can until Dick's son arrives from Lake Tahoe. He is coming down just for an hour because that is about all Dick can handle. Dick cannot speak, and I have to do all the talking and interpreting. It is hard on everyone. Dick does appreciate his son being here, and it is a chance for his son to see how much I care about his father. Overall, it is a good time.

After he leaves, my daughter calls. It has just snowed in Lake Tahoe! They got about three inches and, since it is Memorial Day weekend, it is creating havoc. Everyone arrived with campers, boats, shorts, and sandals, expecting a nice warm weekend by the lake. Instead they got a real snowstorm. I think it sounds exciting and I would love to have been there. It is still hard to give up going to my home I love so much and not being near my children. It is difficult, but it is more important that I be here for Dick.

The rest of the day is quiet and lonely. I realize how much of a closed world I live in. We still get only a few phone calls because no one wants to disturb Dick and no one really understands what is going on in our lives. He is still unable to speak, so I do not hear the sound of his voice, and I try to be quiet for him. It is indeed a very isolated and silent world I am in right now . . . and sometimes very sad.

On the bright side, I am very aware that there is no place I would rather be than beside Dick. I think that says a lot for our relationship.

187

Loneliness

When I cannot feel your warmth beside me
When your arms don't keep me secure
When your touch is missing
I feel lonely.

When I cannot hear your voice
Or see your smile
Or smell your presence
I feel lonely.

When I cannot share what I see
Or feel what I feel
Or hear what I hear with you
I feel lonely.

For the first time in all these years
I have found out the difference
Between being alone and feeling loneliness
And I don't like it.

I will be very lonely without you.
Please don't leave.

5/28 Sunday. Day 89

Today is our anniversary. When we met twenty years ago, I had no idea it would be the best day of my life. Also, I didn't imagine it would lead to a beautiful relationship that would last all these years. I was in a hard place at that time and, I found out later, he was as well.

We met on a flight from San Francisco to New York. I was visiting my mother, and he was continuing on to the Isle of Man for some motorcycle races. Flying on a pass, I wanted to be in first class, but I only got business class. I sat next to him and, because he was talking to someone in first class, I even offered to swap seats (because I knew the cake was better there). He said no. Most of the flight we did not talk. I watched the movie while he read a book: not very eventful. The last half hour, as we were about to land, we started to talk—not about anything special, not about us, just small talk, how I might be looking for job, how he was meeting friends in England. He also spoke of skiing and how good the desserts were on the mountain. I smiled. I thought any man who loved cookies was okay in my book, and that was it. As the plane landed and we were getting off, he asked for my phone numbers in New York and California. He wrote them down on the palm of his hand. Later in the week, as I was walking around New York City, I thought about Dick, and what a gentleman he was—nothing more, just that he was nice.

Back in California, he called and asked me to lunch. I thought it was about a job, so I accepted. Although it was a lovely lunch, there was no job offer and, like before, he shook my hand hello, and again when I left. So much for that.

Shortly thereafter, I flew back to New York to help my brother move to his new home. We were busy moving things from one house to the other, back and forth all day. In the afternoon, the new phone was connected and it rang. My brother answered and said it was for me. I told him it couldn't be because no one knew the new number. He came back again and said it was a call from Europe. I said it couldn't be for me, since I didn't know anyone in Europe. Once more my brother went back to the phone and returned: "He asked for you by name." Finally, I got up and answered the phone.

It was from Dick! How did he ever get the new number? Apparently he had called the old number and it was forwarded to the new one. In the brief conversation, he asked if I would like to join him for lunch. I asked him where he was currently and he replied, "Vienna!" I was blown away! I told him I would think about it, as I was leaving for the airport in about an hour and was supposed to travel on to Miami. I also had to make sure my daughter, who had traveled east with me, got on a flight back to San Francisco.

At the airport, my daughter's 5:00 P.M. flight was delayed and she wasn't able to get on until 5:38 P.M. I said good-bye to her, raced several gates down to the 6:00 P.M. Vienna flight, which was about to leave, and asked if they had a first-class seat available. They said yes, and then I asked if my ticket made out for Miami could be changed. Again, the answer was yes. So with that I raced on board, never looked back, and the rest is history.

On the bright side, thank you, Dick, for all these wonderful years.

190

5/29 Monday. Day 90

Sometimes we all need a good day of rest to regroup. This is one of them. Since it is Memorial Day, we don't have to go to radiation or anywhere else. Dick can sleep, which he needs desperately, and I can relax too. I even have a chance to "play lizard" in the sun. I need it; it is my way of regrouping. I know there is so much I need to do to be caught up, but this is more important. Our nights have been so draining, and we both need some downtime. One thing I have learned from this journey is to prioritize and separate what is really important from what is not. Life has become very basic for me, with getting sleep at the top of the list. Realizing how much good friends and family mean to me are right up there, too. Finding simple things that bring pleasure can make all the difference in the world at the end of the day.

There are no hot dogs, parades, parties, or picnics for us today. We are all alone, and we sleep for hours. Maybe we both know we need our strength for this tough last week ahead.

On the bright side, when Dick is sleeping I can see he is free of pain and torment.

Giving up something you love is hard.

Giving up someone you love is impossible.

All the rest does not matter.

5/30 Tuesday. Day 91

I believe I'm hitting my lowest point today. First, Dick had a horrible night. Accompanied by his usual throat pain, coughing, and spitting out saliva, he now has a terrible nosebleed. We were up all night. He couldn't breathe well and he was coughing constantly. On top of it, I was running around in the wee hours of the morning trying to get the blood off the carpet. Neither one of us had even a halfway decent night's sleep. I am totally worn out and drained.

Then, all day I have been dreading the trip to radiation. I know that with Friday's appointment canceled, and the long holiday weekend, it is imperative for Dick to have his radiation treatment today. I am again holding my breath, and then it happens: he can't do it. He can't breathe while lying down. They call a doctor to see if something could be done, someone comes out to console me, and in the end, it is a total failure. I was devastated.

We go to see Dick's regular radiation doctor, only to be told that he has left, not for the day or week, just left—quit and left. We now have no one familiar with Dick's case. I can hardly hold it together. I know how important this day is. I am not sure whether Dick even cares anymore. He still does not let his feelings out, and I don't know what in the world he is thinking. I am at my wits' end, and it starts to show in front of our favorite nurse. She is very sympathetic but it still doesn't help. She can see the look in my eyes of hopelessness, of despair, of defeat. I look up and say I am just tired. We leave with the understanding that now Dick will have to add another day to his treatment to make up for this missed one. We will have to come back through next Monday.

I was so hoping this would be over. Where am I going to find the strength? I am so fragile now. Where do I find my positive attitude I need to help Dick through this? It has all disappeared. I feel so lost.

We continue back to the hospital in silence so he can have his blood work done to be ready for chemo tomorrow. I don't go in. For the first time, I am not by Dick's side. I just can't be. I need space. I drive around and pick him up when he is done. We drive home in silence. It is silent still. There is nothing to say.

On the bright side, we got a nice card from the owners of Has Beans with two lotto tickets inside. I lost there, too.

194

5/31 Wednesday. Day 92

It's the last day of the month and what more can go wrong? How can things go from terrible to impossible so quickly? I should have known today would be one of those days: it is Wednesday, the day I hate the most. Dick and I are silent all morning. I am still upset. I know I should not take it out on him, but I am just so frustrated with him for being unable to do his radiation treatment. I know he is having a hard time and he has claustrophobia, but he is so close to the end.

It begins with a trip to the hospital for his weekly chemotherapy treatment. Once we are in the infusion room, Dick is told they will not start the IV of Erbitux until his chemotherapy doctor comes in to see him—definitely not a good way to begin the day. I figure the doctor has heard about Dick's difficult time at radiation yesterday and wants to see what is going on in his throat. We wait for an hour before she comes in. That was hard enough, but then she decides to halt his chemotherapy because the inside of Dick's throat is so raw and filled with blisters. She cancels his treatment.

I can't believe it! He has only one more week after this for his chemotherapy. I know he badly needs it, as it will help with the radiation treatments. With his cancer in stage 4, Dick needs every bit of help he can get. She also cancels the treatment for next week. We leave defeated and have just enough time to drive to radiation.

At radiation things are not much better. Dick is again having a hard time lying down without choking. A new doctor is called and tells the technicians to do whatever it takes but to get his radiation treatment completed. They decide not to put the upper and lower trays in his mouth, and not to use the block of wood that holds his mouth in the right position. He finally gets through it. I just hope they were able to hit the right spot. On the way home, Dick expresses to me he is beginning to feel his claustrophobia again and he doesn't think he can do any more.

All in all, it is an exhausting day. I spend the evening eating and crying by myself. I am so drained. A girlfriend calls and hears how badly I am doing and immediately calls someone she knows who is a caregiver and can more easily understand the desperation in my voice. A few minutes later that person calls and talks to me. I guess it helps. It is at least nice to be able to communicate with someone who understands the language and the process I am going through. All your friends are willing to help. But they really understand very little about this situation, unless they have been through it. Overall, it is an impossible day.

On the bright side, there are only three more radiation treatments to go.

How Much More Can I Hurt?

How much more can I possibly hurt?
How much more can seep out from me
without leaving me numb?
How much more can the little slings and arrows sting
without burning?
How much more can I continually keep giving
without getting back?
How much longer can I keep going
without needing comfort for myself?
How much more disappointment and sadness
can my heart hold without breaking?
How much more can I possibly give
when everything I have has already been given?
And tell me, how much more can I hurt
without falling apart?

June

June

6/1 Thursday. Day 93

Out of all the days so far, this has to be the worst. How can I say that after yesterday? Regardless, it's a new low for me. When I get up this morning, after another night of little sleep for either one of us, Dick gets his pad and starts to write. I know it has to be something important for him to try to write, especially so early in the morning.

He writes, "I don't want you to be mad at me but I can't go to radiation. I just can't do it anymore." I am devastated. I try to explain how very important this last little bit is, but he is determined. He points to his head and tries to write out the word *claustrophobia*. I get the message. Once Dick feels this way, nothing is going to change his mind.

All morning I wait to see if he will get better, but it does not happen. Finally, I give up and say I will go to radiation and talk to everyone involved and tell them what has occurred. I am so drained I can hardly move.

As soon as I walk in the door, everyone knows something is wrong. The nice nurse, Jill, sees me first and asks what has happened. Besides my being there at the wrong time, she can see Dick is not with me, and can definitely see the look on my face. I lose it and tears fill up my eyes. She takes me aside and we talk. She explains that of all the cancers to treat, throat cancer is the hardest on the patient, and it is horribly tough to get through. She says she saw it coming and I cry all over again. She tells me he had excellent care, he had tried his best, I had done a wonderful job, and that was all I could do. I feel like such a failure. I need to be able to do more, and I just cannot find what it might be. We discuss making a follow-up appointment in a few weeks. I say I will, but first I want to say good-bye to the technicians in radiation.

Walking down the hall, I am a mess. It is going to be difficult to face the people who have tried so hard to help Dick through his treatments. I talk with Amanda, who hugs me and is kind. I say I'm sorry and she understands. We say good-bye and hug again. Back down the hall another technician comes up to me and sees the look on my face, and we go through it all over again, tears and hugs. When will this ever end?

I make a follow-up appointment and leave. There is nothing more I can do. There is nothing at all—nothing inside me, no hope, no dreams, no beliefs, no promises, and no future. There aren't even any more tears; they are all drained too. It is a very lonely drive home, aside from the fact that I am in the car by myself.

Later, I tell Dick I love him and we will have to go on from here. I change his bandage as I have done every day since his feeding tube was inserted and make sure he is comfortable. Later that night, after I have finished talking and crying to my daughters, another call comes in. It is from the radiation doctor who saw Dick yesterday. He urges me to try to get Dick back to finish his treatments. I can't believe it. Could there be any hope after all? I immediately tell Dick about the call. He doesn't want to discuss it but motions that we will talk about it tomorrow.

On the bright side, there will be a tomorrow and I see Dovie's new baby for the first time. Thank you, Jill, Amanda, and Hernando, for all your compassion.

Where Do You Go?

Where do you go when hope begins to fade?
When the lights dim and all your strength starts to ebb?
Where do you go to be reassured?
Where do you go to feel safe and secure?
Where do you go in the middle of the night
when you feel so alone?
Where do you go to find some peace?
Or even a place where you can yell out loud?
Where is that warm, fuzzy blanket when you need it?
And most of all, where are all the answers?
Please tell me, where do you go?

6/2 Friday. Day 94

The radiation doctor who called last night wanted Dick at radiation today no matter what. I'd said I would try to talk to him. This morning Dick writes and asks me if he has a doctor appointment.

Puzzled, I ask, "What do you mean? Radiation is over because you said you couldn't do it."

He now scribbles down that he wants to try, but wants to find an alternative to the mask, maybe being anesthetized or something along that line.

I call radiation. After talking with several people, I am told Dick's mask has been thrown out. They will have to make a new one. I realize it won't work because it took Dick two different days to have the mask fitted the first time. The heat of the material on his face made him extremely claustrophobic, and there is no way he will be able to go through it again.

I told Dick and he writes, "Call the doctor back and leave a message to explain I am willing to try again, except the mask has been thrown out and the file closed." I leave a nice message on the machine and thank the doctor for his effort anyway.

So much for tomorrow being a better day . . . shit. Now Dick is depressed and I am stressed out. Am I the one who failed him by going to radiation yesterday?

Dick is not doing at all well mentally today, so I stay near. I have been watching for this to occur. Sooner or latter he had to realize the gravity of the situation. I think it is now sinking in. He even takes off his Lance Armstrong "Live Forever" bracelet. I tell him we must deal with the situation and go on from here. I mention some advanced new procedures I have heard of that we can discuss down the road. I reassure him and am as supportive as I am capable of being. We hold hands and comfort each other. As always, I tell him I loved him, very, very much.

And then it happens. Radiation calls and says they have found Dick's mask and want him to come up right then! It is already 5:00 P.M. and they close at 6:00 P.M. I talk to Dick and know there is no way he can prepare himself mentally this fast. Also, we would not make it through the traffic in time. I tell the assistant he has just taken medicine and is asleep. We agree he will return on Monday.

Wow, what a reversal. This roller-coaster ride is mentally very exhausting. Maybe there is some hope after all. At least Dick will have the weekend to settle down.

The other good news is that my daughters are coming down to give me help and support. They say they will drop everything, drive down, and meet me for dinner in a few hours! I feel like a baby who can't take care of myself. Perhaps it is what I need right now, both physically and mentally. Suddenly, my spirits are up. I tell Dick and he gives me the thumbs-up. I can tell he sees how much it means to me. The roller coaster is going up hill again.

On the bright side, I am positive again and looking forward to the weekend. Also, I will get to show my granddaughter the new baby bird!

6/3 Saturday. Day 95

It was wonderful to go out and meet my daughters last night, especially since I haven't been out for dinner in so many months. Dick and I don't sit together while I eat because the smell of food continues to be difficult for him. Also, it causes him to be more depressed, and of course there is no conversation. He simply has his cans of nutrition while I eat alone. So it was very good to get out and I was looking forward to a happy weekend.

The original idea today is to have my daughters go shopping and help me buy sheets for our bed. Dick spends so much time in it that I need another set. Instead, we get sidetracked going to garage sales. We have a wonderful, lighthearted time, even with me checking my cell phone constantly to see if Dick has dialed my number. Though he can't speak, we have an agreement that if his number shows up on my phone, he needs me, and I will immediately come home. Also, I never travel more than a mile or two from our house.

The afternoon is spent lounging by the pool at our complex with my granddaughter, Mylie. Since they all live at Lake Tahoe and it is not as warm there this time of year, swimming is something new to her. In the end, my daughters lounge while I spend the whole time in the water with Mylie. We all have a wonderful time! It is so good for me to relax and good for my daughters to see me that way, too. They are as worried for me as they are for Dick. Eventually, we leave and accomplish our mission to buy the sheets, having dinner out so as not to disturb Dick.

By evening, we are tired but manage to play cards and still laugh. That laughter is good for all of us.

On the bright side, everything is bright and I had a very good day. Also, there are two baby birds, not one, in the nest. I will show my granddaughter tomorrow.

6/4 Sunday. Day 96

It is supposed to be a late morning but Mylie wakes early and begins playing, which ends any sleep for the rest of us. Tammy and Robin help clean the house, organize the refrigerator, do laundry, vacuum, and, most important, help change the bed to make Dick more comfortable. Dick sits outside while some of this is going on so the dust and commotion will not get to him. He is in more of a fog these days, and the less turmoil, the better. Mylie is good too; she watches a DVD. Having a clean house not only helps me catch up physically, but also enables me mentally to feel organized and better able to focus on the important things, like Dick.

Then it is off to the pool again. The girls have hay fever that is not letting up. It is hard to see them suffer. Finally it is time for them to leave. After all, they have husbands and a world of their own. They make food for me (to make sure I will eat), pack up their stuff, and leave. All in all it has been a wonderful day for me. I got a chance to get away from what is going on in my head, and it was fun playing with my granddaughter in the pool. I, like most grandparents, wish their children lived closer. I never thought I would be the one to say it, though.

Later my girlfriend calls; we had talked on Friday and she had been very troubled when I mentioned what occurred in radiation. I say I hadn't meant to get her upset, and maybe we should not talk about cancer at all. She disagrees. We decide to make plans to do a few things together when my life has calmed down. Sometimes I forget when I discuss cancer with others that it can be quite foreign and frightening to them. They become uncomfortable, as it is not their world. I remember I was this way in the beginning, but it is my world now and seems almost "normal." Who would ever think I would say that word when speaking about cancer?

———————————

On the bright side, where do I start? Having a great weekend with Tammy, Robin, and Mylie has made my world complete and has enabled me to regroup. I also got to show my granddaughter Dovie and her babies!

6/5 Monday. Day 97

How did I know this is going to happen? Actually, I did. After a wonderful weekend with my "girls" I have the rug pulled out from under me. Last night Dick experienced the worst night ever. He couldn't get his coughing and saliva under control. We got up and settled him on the living room couch. It was the first time Dick and I did not sleep together. He insisted I should get some rest, even if he could not. So neither one of us slept. For me, it was because I can tell the roller coaster I am on is about to take a dive. I know I had too good of a weekend and had been away from this cancer too long.

It starts this morning when I ask Dick if he is going to be able to go to radiation, as we are expected there. Then the crash happens head-on: he writes "No." No, he can't do it or no, he won't do it, it doesn't matter. The result is the same. It is over. He has had enough, and when Dick makes up his mind, nothing is going to change it.

I try everything. I call radiation and talk to the nurse, who in turn talks to the doctor. Dick is prescribed Ativan to calm him down. I know it won't do any good. He has tried it before with no success. Dick's mind is made up. Between the choking on the saliva when he lies down for the treatment, and the claustrophobia of the mask, he is not going to do it. He won't even try. He is angry with me for even suggesting it. He writes down that the way he feels now, he couldn't even get his motorcycle helmet on. He is not in a good mood and his throat hurts more than ever.

I give up. I accept the AA saying about how there are some things you can change, some things you cannot, and you need the wisdom to know the difference. I finally get the wisdom. It is over. No more radiation and no more chemotherapy. We will have to see where we go from here. I call radiation back and cancel today's treatment.

The rest of the day doesn't go well either. I tell Dick I need to be away from him for a while. I say I don't want to be mad at him and regret it later. I do not want it as a memory. I stay in another bedroom and write most of the day. Dick actually drives the car to the post office by himself — a first in months. I think he is relieved since he doesn't have to go to radiation, and he feels he can do anything.

I call a girlfriend and have her come over after work so I can get out all I have inside me. I explain that I don't want to take it out on Dick but it is hard. It feels good to talk it out and she is supportive. I am so very lucky to be able to have someone to call. I wish Dick had someone. I even suggest later that he needs to talk to somebody, and he doesn't say no. Maybe tomorrow I will be able to deal with this. For the rest of today, I am just too drained and sad. I feel that I have failed Dick and this is a turning point in his treatment. I think Dick realizes it too, because he seems very quiet most of the day.

On the bright side, the decision has been made, and that was the hardest part.

6/6 Tuesday. Day 98

Today starts off poorly. Dick did not sleep well on the couch last night. He is very tired and sleeps most of the day. We are both very drained as we near the end of these first one hundred days.

A friend comes over and picks up our second car to sell for us. He wants to know how much I want for it. I tell him I just need less to worry about. The price isn't so important—even though we could use the money, as neither one of us is working. Once again, I am reminded of the quote I wrote a while ago about what is really important in life. Dick loves the car, but he is not driving now. We will see what the future holds. I tell Dick we can always get another car after he feels better.

Afterward, I have a difficult experience about which I do not care to write. Although I am quite open with my own emotions, I would never want to hurt anyone else's feelings. So I go out and buy some flowers to plant instead. Gardening always takes my mind off things. It is the best therapy for me besides writing. Anyone who becomes a caregiver needs to have some sort of outlet to relieve his or her own stress. We will be going to see the chemotherapy doctor tomorrow, and I do not want to think about any decision that may be made.

Later, Chris comes over and we have a glass of wine together. She teaches me to play a new card game. She makes me feel better.

On the bright side, Kathy left some food at my door this morning and a bright yellow sunflower. What a thoughtful thing to do. She is very special, too.

6/7 Wednesday. Day 99

We go to see the chemotherapy doctor today. Dick is being dismissed. There is nothing more they can do for him. The last two sessions have been canceled because his throat is so bad. We will just have to wait and see what the main oncology doctor says next week.

That should be a heavy day. I am not looking forward to it. I am not sure it will be good news. There is so much uncertainty about this whole journey. Not much is told to you along the way. The reasoning is that too much information can be very unnerving and depressing. The doctor says it is because it would be overwhelming to take it all in and much too hard to understand. Besides, when doctors say "difficult" they mean "impossible," and when they say "discomfort" they mean "extreme pain." It is a whole different language to comprehend. I have learned that much.

It is hard to be discharged from the chemotherapy doctor since she is the only one we have even seen halfway regularly. At least we have a few days to rest and regroup. Dick really needs it, too. We both have been getting less than five hours' sleep each night, and I don't see it getting better until the end of next week.

He is now seven days out from his last radiation treatment. We have been told it takes at least two weeks before he will start feeling better. I am counting the seconds.

———————————

On the bright side, the baby birds are getting bigger, and they are fun to watch. Also, I am happy we do not have to go to see any doctors until next week. I will have a few days to prepare myself.

6/8 Thursday. Day 100

Finally, we have a good day. We are free of the commitments of cancer—not cancer itself, but at least for a few days we do not have to go anywhere or do anything cancer-related. We can simply take care of ourselves. It is also the hundredth day of this journey—a milestone, so to speak. Not that I ever wanted to be in the position of keeping track like this. It is what it is: one hundred days and counting.

This is also the beginning of getting out of the house. Dick insists I join our motorcycle club for a dinner function on the other side of the bay. He can't go, since he can't eat, drink, or speak, but he wants me to get out and rejoin the rest of the world. I don't want to go, but he thinks it will be good for me. And it is.

First, I stop in Sausalito to visit a girlfriend I haven't seen in quite a while. Before today, I had not been able to get away for this long. I even convince her to join me for the dinner.

Second, everyone at the motorcycle club dinner is very nice to me, caring and concerned about Dick. Most club members hadn't realized how much he's been through, but they send their best wishes anyway. It is good to for me to relay the news to Dick. Cancer patients are still aware of the outside world, even when they are not able to participate. Hearing about it helps them to live in less of an isolated cocoon.

Third, Dick has gotten out again today. It is good for his confidence. He goes to Has Beans and sits and reads the paper. He can't talk, but the owners are very nice to him and he feels comfortable. It is important for him to feel "normal" and realize he will again be able to do things for himself. The first wave of treatments is drawing to a close, and hopefully, he will feel better in a few weeks.

Lastly, tonight as I am on the phone talking with my daughter, Dick does something that means more to me than anything else. I am telling Tammy how much I miss my granddaughter and the way she spoke the word "Beautiful" when I last saw her. Repeatedly I say the word as she said it: "Bee-u-tee-full," pronouncing every syllable. It is so precious. Passing by the room, Dick comes over and pokes me several times. I try to ask what he wants, but he just pokes me again.

"What do you want?" I say and go back to my conversation. He again pokes me. I look at my shoulder and ask, "Sunburn?" No, that isn't it.

Finally, exasperated, I tell him I am on the phone with Tammy; he pokes once again and mouths the words, "You are beautiful."

What more can I say? My world is so complete with him. I need nothing more. This is indeed a very good day.

On the bright side, it was beautiful seeing Sausalito and all the boats. Thank you, Sally B.; and many thanks, Chris and Gene, for making us feel so comfortable at Has Beans. Best of all, today was the day Dovie's babies left the nest—a new beginning for all!

Conclusion

The first one hundred days and nights are finally over. It has been a long haul. Cancer isn't over. It is now a way of life, but the initial shock and treatments are finished.

From here there will be many more days and nights of roller-coaster emotions, the very highs and the very lows. This is far from the end, but at least we have a better idea of what is involved. The first wave of treatments—chemotherapy and radiation—is finished, as much as Dick was able to do. Now we are in the system and understand how it works. We know the terms to use and are familiar with the places we have to go. We are better able to work with different doctors, nurses, staff, and all the other people involved along this journey. Now we are equipped to ask the right questions and get the correct information. The initial shock has worn off, even if it has worn us down.

There will be time for Dick to recuperate. There will be time for me, too. There will be time to read and understand more about this cancer and cancer options; time to get caught up with the outside world and with friends who had to stay at a distance; time with my daughters to enjoy their company and their pregnancies; and time to put our house in order, literally. Maybe there will even be time to sleep and become human again. I've always known that time is precious, but now it is even more so. And I will enjoy the sun on my face with extra zest and smell the flowers I love so much with deeper intensity. I will feel all that life has to offer to the utmost—every moment.

Although I still think in days, and sometimes even in mo-

ments, at least there are times I can think in weeks. Weeks between doctor appointments, blood tests, and all that happens
with follow-up treatments. I do not plan ahead, but I am beginning to think ahead. Maybe we will be able to go to the mountains, or maybe Dick will be strong enough to do this or that...
Still, it is like the lull before a storm, and I know this storm is
brewing. The doctor has already told us he would build Dick up
only to tear him down again. Those were his exact words. I
heard them, even if Dick didn't. The doctor wants Dick to go
through an operation to have his lymph nodes removed when
he is stronger. He already looked me in the eye and reminded
me the statistics still aren't very good.

There will never be freedom from cancer. I know that is not
a possibility. The world we live in at this time is filled with terms
such as *remission, cancer survivor, probabilities,* and *percentages.* I
don't think of these either. It would be wasted energy. I cannot
change what will be. I can only deal with what we have, and I
will.

There are places I do not think about visiting now. I have no
desire to. I don't think in years but take each day, week, and
month as it comes. I don't think of what if, what could have
been, or what should be. I do not dwell on time lost, but rather
on time I have gained. It is like looking at a glass of water that is
either half full or half empty, all depending on one's outlook.
My glass is half full, and I will make the most of it.

For now, I will take it as I find it, a moment at a time, a day
to regroup, and a week for Dick to get stronger. I cannot think
further ahead or hope for too much. I will not be greedy. I am
very grateful for all I have at this moment. Dick will get better,
at least for a while, before the next storm. I am not sure he sees
it, but I do. Each day there is a little hint of hope and a little more
brightness.

Our time is more precious than ever, and I will relish every
moment Dick and I have together. My touch will be more sensi-

tive, my love more profound. I have Dick for now, and *now* is the place I want to be.

I will not look at the future. It is still too hard. I already know there is so much more Dick and I must endure.

The rest of our lives together will be filled with follow-up doctor's appointments, more surgeries, and more recovery periods. For now, I will take each day with an appreciation of that time only—one more day with Dick, one more day of life.

I will be there every step of the way for Dick, no matter how long or short this journey may be. I will build up my strength again and be ready for all there is to come. I will be strong for both of us. I have to be. I have been his friend and constant companion all these years, and now his wife too. Nothing will change. I will be Dick's sentry dove, watching over him with protection and love. I am his caregiver, and that is the most important role I have ever had. I will be there

for all there is to come,

with all I have in me,

with all that I am.

—*Gloria Burola McSorley, Caregiver*

Part Two

Practical Advice
and Useful Hints

Tips for Caregivers

Caregivers can make an enormous difference in a cancer patient's recovery. Whether going to the doctor, offering words of encouragement, or nursing through the rough times, supportive caregivers can be the best ally, personal cheerleader, and advocate, as well as a life preserver when most needed.

Caregivers shoulder a big responsibility. It is the ultimate endurance test. Supporting patients through an aggressive program of cancer treatment can be twenty-four hours a day, seven days a week —an emotional, draining job. A caregiver is an essential part of the overall health-care team, working closely with doctors and nurses to assist with medications, home care, and feeding. Yet caregivers and their needs are largely overlooked by the health-care system.

Caregivers can feel just as stressed and overwhelmed as patients. Research has shown that caregivers can even suffer physical and emotional problems. As people who already have the responsibility of a family, a job, and a full life, now they have the additional task of caregiving. There may be times when caregivers will feel angry, resentful, frustrated, overwhelmed, and then guilty for feeling all those emotions. It is normal to react this way. Cancer is a scary, unwanted intruder in everyone's world.

Hopefully, the following tips will include some things that a caregiver can do to make the task easier.

Take care of yourself first. It is easy to forget, when you are taking care of someone else, that you need care too. Think of your own health and well-being. Do not feel guilty for thinking about your own needs. It is crucial to take care of yourself. The cancer patient is getting care, but if you don't take care of yourself, no one else will. You will more likely be able to avoid health problems, to have more energy and enthusiasm while caring for the cancer patient, and to generally feel better about yourself.

Take time for yourself. Time is the most important thing to remember when caring for your own well-being. Caregivers need to know it is all right to take some time off. Schedule some time for yourself. You need a break to attend to personal needs or to relax. If you are exhausted and stressed, you cannot give the best care to the patient. Arrange for someone else to take over your caregiving duties temporarily.

Prioritize your time. Decide to cope with only what is most important. Delegate or leave undone the rest. Plan time each day to be alone, to regroup and rest, both emotionally and physically, a time when the cancer patient does not need you. Trade time with another caregiver. If possible, find a caregiver to swap time with for a morning or afternoon off.

Acknowledge your limitations and reach out for help. No matter how strong you may think you are, you can use help. Ask friends and family, relatives, church members, coworkers, members of social or athletic organizations you belong to, or neighbors to lend a hand. Keep a good contact list of all those who are able to help, what they can do, and times they are available. Be prepared to ask them to fulfill specific tasks. Ask if they can set up a regular schedule an hour or two a week to help out.

Take care of your health. Eat a healthy diet. When you are busy caring for others, remember to take the time to maintain your own nutritional needs, so you can keep your energy level up each day.

Get some exercise, even if just for a few minutes. As tired as you can become, a few moments a day can actually boost your energy level and can help relieve stress.

Recognize stress and take precautions to manage it.

Remember to recharge your emotional batteries as well, to cope better with your fears, worries, and concerns.

Turn to the cancer society.

Turn to a national volunteer support group, Website, or books; just turn somewhere.

You will find that help will come to you and you'll learn to cope somehow, someway. If all else fails, turn to your inner self for strength.

And if finances allow:

- Hire a teenager, older adult, church member, or friend to stay with the cancer patient for a few hours each day.
- Hire a cleaning service to help out around the house, and use that time as your own regrouping time.
- Set up a schedule for a home delivery meal service at least once a week.
- Hire a professional home health aide.

Overall, the idea is to make life as easy and uncomplicated as possible for yourself, so you are better able to focus and deal with your loved one through this cancer journey.

Things to Do for a Caregiver

Friends and family often want to be of assistance through hard times but don't know how best to help. When friends or relatives call and ask if they can do anything, the offer is often vague. What is "anything"? When is the right time? How much are they willing to do? Make a list of the things you really need. Friends and family can sign up for specific tasks. Be direct and straightforward. This can be a source of relief to you as well as to them. The following are a few suggestions where others may be of assistance.

Food

- Accompany you to grocery store and unload groceries.
- Take the grocery list, go shopping for you, and unload them at home. prepare a box of healthy snacks or finger foods ready to eat. plan a week's worth of dinners.
- Help schedule friends and family members to cook for you and your family; each can make one meal a day for later use. (Remember to deliver meals in marked containers that can be returned easily.)

Transportation

- Take patient to doctor appointments.
- Take patient to and from the hospital.
- Take children to and from school and activities.

Run errands

- Go to the cleaners, video store, grocery store.
- Go to the pharmacy to pick up prescriptions.

At home

- Do general house cleaning: laundry, dishes, dust, vacuum.
- Offer to baby-sit.
- Work in the yard.
- Cut the grass.
- Water the lawn, water the plants.
- Wash a car.
- Be on call for unexpected problems (handyman for broken car, leaking faucets, etc.).
- Walk the dog.

Be a secretary for a day

- Return phone calls from messages on answering machine.
- Offer to keep everyone apprised of developments.
- Help pay bills and keep track of insurance papers, etc.
- Help with all medical paperwork and keep it organized.
- Read through all the cancer information and consolidate it.

Give a caregiver time off in any way possible. And above all, listen and be a shoulder to lean on when needed.

This is what I wanted during my difficult times (your needs may be different):

Please Do

- Please bring me flowers I can plant and not cut flowers that will die in a week.
- Do cater a meal for me or bring in food you made yourself. I am too tired to cook.
- Do make a calendar and gather friends to sign up for different days to do things.
- Do hire a cleaning person one day a month or more. I will use that time for myself.
- Do offer to be a secretary for a day, to pay my bills, make phone calls, or solve problems.
- Do be an errand runner, or gardener or day-care provider for a day or more.
- Do give me my favorite wine. Sooner or later I will have a chance to drink it.
- Do give me a certificate for a manicure, or haircut, massage or a trip to a day spa.
- Do anything to make me feel feminine and human.
- Do read through all the cancer information I have collected and consolidate it. Please do because my brain cannot think anymore!

Things for a Cancer Patient

Even if the person suffering from cancer is too ill to see you, there are things you can offer them that will be appreciated. Here are a few:

- Cards to let them know they are not forgotten and are thought about.
- A portable DVD player to distract them while going through chemotherapy treatments.
- Books on subjects that interest them, crosswords, etc.
- A new set of sheets, since the patient will spend a lot of time resting.
- A gift basket filled with useful items like small notebook and pen, whiteboard, marker, and eraser if they are not able to speak.
- Post-It notes.
- Certificates that can be used as time allows such as a day trip to a spa, a haircut, a massage, nails done, anything to help them feel human.
- Certificate for a cleaning person to come in one day a month or more.
- Book of coupons made by friends for different responsibilities and tasks.

What I Have Learned

Throughout this journey as a cancer caregiver there has been a great deal I have learned. Here are some things I have found that helped both the cancer patient and the caregiver.

1. *Doctor's appointments*

- When going to an appointment, go prepared. A doctor's time is limited, and it is best to make the most of this time.
- Have a special notebook to organize all your medical information, medical records, doctor information, operations, appointments, chemotherapy and radiation information, etc., and especially a list of names, phone numbers of doctors, medications, etc. (See the Sample Forms section below.) Bring the notebook with you to appointments. Include a list of questions you have written down beforehand so you will be better organized and not forget something you wanted to ask. Make them specific and brief, and ask your most important questions first. Do not be ashamed of "dumb" questions. This is a new world you are entering, and it will take some time to understand everything there is to know.
- Write down notes about the doctor says and any instructions that need to be followed for future reference.
- Keep a calendar to be able to coordinate appointments better.
- Keep a diary of symptoms, such as when, what, weight loss, etc., to better aid the doctor in your treatment and care. (See

Sample Forms.)

- Doctors need to understand your needs and concerns. It is important to have a good relationship with your doctors. They need to take the time to listen to your concerns and help you get answers to your questions. Sometimes too much information is hard to handle all at once. Do not be afraid to speak up and tell your doctor how much or how little information you want at one time. It may be that you just want simple directions about what pill to take, or you may want to know a lot of medical details about your illness. Sometimes, without realizing it, doctors will use terms you don't understand. Ask your doctor to translate and explain anything you do not comprehend. Ask the doctor to rephrase information to make it easier for you to understand. They are usually very willing to explain. It makes their job easier if a patient can follow instructions clearly.

- When visiting the doctor or at other encounters with the medical establishment, try to have a family member or friend accompany the patient, to help with support and to remember what was said. When one hears difficult news, one often experiences shock and doesn't hear much else. Take time to digest what is happening and to understand.

- Also bring something to do while waiting for appointments. It makes the time easier to pass, distracts your mind from where you are, and can even give you some time to organize some of the other parts of your life. If you are unable to have someone with you, ask the doctor if you can use a tape recorder so you won't forget anything later.

2. *At home*

- Have one location in the home where you keep all the medical information, insurance papers, telephone numbers, and one notebook with all the information you take with you to appointments. This way you will be able to locate information easily.

- Use Post-It notes on cabinets or anywhere you are likely to notice them to help keep track of all that needs to be done. When you are exhausted it is easy to forget important details. Let others see them and let them help where they can. (I found this very helpful, as friends could see special tasks I needed done and they could offer to fulfill those specific needs.)

3. *Know your resources*

- Talk to anyone you can to get the information you need to help you and the cancer patient get through these tough times. Talk with hospital social workers about patient assistance programs, transportation help, support groups, and financial support. Use the resource lists at the back of this book. Do not try to cope with this alone, as it becomes overwhelming. Also, research all you can on new developments. Remember that correct information is the most valuable tool you can have.

4. *Have a support network*

- Become a one-person support group of your own for the cancer patient.
- Have a friend to lean on, dump on, or cry on.
- Seek out caregiver and/or patient support groups in your community.

Above all, the most important thing is good and open communication among the cancer patient, the caregiver, the doctors, the nurses, the medical technicians, etc. Usually people with cancer want and need understanding, not sympathy, and realistic help, not overindulgence.

Sample Forms

TELEPHONE NUMBERS

NAME _____   _____ MR#

DOCTOR	TELEPHONE NO.	ADDRESS

BODY CHART

NAME _____   _____ MR#

	Date	Blood Pressure	Weight	Temperature	Heart Rate	Pulse	Other
1							
2							
3							
4							
5							
6							
7							
8							
9							
10							
11							
12							
13							
14							
15							
16							
17							
18							
19							
20							
21							
22							
23							
24							
25							
26							
27							
28							

MEDICINE CHART

NAME _____   _____ MR#

	Medicine	Amount	Dose	For	Time	Side Effects	Doctor
1							
2							
3							
4							
5							
6							
7							
8							
9							
10							
11							
12							
13							
14							
15							
16							
17							
18							
19							
20							

Titles of Poems and Random Quotes

Books about Caregivers and Caregiving

Abramson, Alexis *The Caregiver's Survival Handbook: How to Care for Your Aging Parent without Losing Yourself*

Adler, Karen Kirzner, Kleiman, Rozlyn *Cancer Caregivers—A Resource Guide*

American Cancer Society, *Cancer Caregiving A–Z: An At-Home Guide for Patients and Families*

Brown, Pamela N. *Facing Cancer Together: How to Help Your Friend or Loved One*

Clark, Elizabeth J. ed., *Teamwork: The Cancer Patient's Guide to Talking with Your Doctor* (A publication of the National Coalition for Cancer Survivorship)

Daneker, Bonnie Bajorek *The Compassionate Caregiver's Guide to Caring for Someone with Cancer*

Davis, Lorraine Valyo *I Need to Scream! Would Anyone Even Hear Me? (A Personal Caregiver's Survival Guide)*

Hennessey, Maya *If Only I'd Had This Caregiving Book*

Hobson, Alan, Hobson, Cecilia *Climb Back from Cancer: A Survivor and Caregiver's Inspirational Journey*

Hoults, Peter, Bucher, Julia American Cancer Society, *Caregiving: A Step-by-Step Resource for Caring for the Person with Cancer at Home*

Jacobs, Barry J. *The Emotional Survival Guide for Caregivers: Looking after Yourself and Your Family While Helping an Aging Parent*

Keim, Rachel, Smith, Ginny *What to Eat Now: The Cancer Lifeline Cookbook and Easy-to-Use Nutrition Guide to Delicious and Healthy Eating for Cancer Patients, Survivors, and Caregivers*

Molloy, Kevin *Cancer: How Will I Get Through This? Stories of Hope from Survivors and Caregivers*

National Family Caregivers Association, *The Resourceful Caregiver: Helping Family Caregivers Help Themselves*

Pedicone, Wendi Fox *Hanging Out with Lab Coats: Hope, Humor & Help for Cancer Patients and Their Caregivers*

Resources

About Face: www.aboutfaceusa.org Oral, head, and neck care

American Association of Retired People: 800-424-3410
www.aarp.org/caregiving
Caregiving/Family support/Older persons

American Cancer Society (ACS): 800-ACS-2345
www.cancer.org
General resources/Insurance/Financial assistance

American Cancer Society
      After Diagnosis
      Understanding Radiation Therapy
      Understanding Chemotherapy
      Listen With Your Heart
      Talking With Your Doctor
      Nutrition for the Person with Cancer
      Nausea and Vomiting
      Caring for the Patient with Cancer at Home
      Advanced Cancer and Palliative Care

American Society of Clinical Oncology: 703-299-0150
www.asco.org
A leading cancer organization for the scientific and education exchange and an active advocate on behalf of cancer patients and their health-care providers.

Cancer Care: 800-813-HOPE www.cancercare.org
General resources/Patient support

Cancer Hope Network: 877-467-3638
www.cancerhopenetwork.org
Patient support

Cancer Information Service (National Cancer Institute): 800-422-6897 www.cancer.gov
General resources

Cancer Research and Prevention Foundation: 800-227-2732
www.preventcancer.org
Prevention/Research

Cancer Survival Toolbox: 877-866-5748
www.cancersurvicaltoolbox.org
A free audio resource program (10 tapes, half hour to an hour and a half each)

Caregivers, Inc.: 800-829-2734 www.caregiver.com Provides an online newsletter, workshops, audio tapes, information on caregivers and the workforce, caregiver tips, and other topics.

Mettler, Molly, MSW and Kemper, Donald W. MPH Community Hospital of the Monterey Peninsula Healthwise Publications *Healthwise for Life: Your Resource for Healthy Living*

Family Caregiver Alliance (FCA): 800-445-8106
www.caregiver.org
Caregiving/Family support

Glucksberg, Harold M.D., Singer, Jack W., M.D. *Cancer Care: A Personal Guide*, John Hopkins University Press

Harpham, Wendy Schlessel, M.D. *Diagnosis Cancer: Your Guide Through The First Few Months*

Holleb, Arthur I., M.D., ed. *The American Cancer Society Cancer Book: Prevention, Detection, Diagnosis, Treatment, Rehabilitation, Cure*

Houts, Peter S., ed. *American College of Physicians Home Care Guide for Cancer for Family and Friends Giving Care at Home*

Lance Armstrong Foundation: 512-236-8820 www.laf.org Education/Research

Lange, Vladimir, M.D. *Be a Survivor: Your Guide to Breast Cancer Treatment*

Let's Face It: 360-676-7325 www.faceit.org Oral, head, and neck care

Medicare (Caregivers information page): www.medicare.gov/caregivers

National Alliance for Caregiving: www.caregiving.org

National Cancer Institute (NCI): 800-422-6897 www.cancer.gov, www.cancernet.nci.nih.gov Research and information/Clinical trials
>   *What you need to know about Cancer of the Esophagus*
>   *What you need to know abut Oral Cancer*
>   *Chemotherapy and You: A Guide to Self-Help during Cancer Treatment*

National Coalition for Cancer Survivorship: 877-NCCS-YES
(622-7937) www.canceradvocacy.org
General and online resources/Programs and publications

National Family Caregivers Association: www.nfcacares.org
800-896-3650
Family support

Oncology Nursing Society: 888-257-4667 www.ond.org,
www.asco.org
A variety of educational publications, audiovisual materials,
and annual conferences.

Schimmel, Selma R. with Barry Fox. M.D.*Cancer Talk: Voices of
Hope and Endurance from "The Group Room" the World's Largest
Cancer Support Group*

Support for People with Oral, Head, and Neck Cancer: 800-
377-0928 www.spohnc.org

Strength for Caring: 888-ICARE80
www.StrengthForCaring.com Provides caregivers with knowledge and tools needed to better understand cancer and cancer
treatments, managing the patient's symptoms, dealing with
changing family roles, tapping community resources, and improving the caregiver's physical and mental health. A free program taught by nurses and social workers.

Trotti, III, Andy M.D. *Side Effects of Head and Neck Cancer Treatment: Practical Guide to Mouth Sores and Dry Mouth*

The Wellness Community: 888-793-9355
www.wellness-community.org

Additional Web Sites:
www.caregiving.com
www.cancer.org
www.cancercarecenter.com 888-721-9369
www.canceradvocacy.org 877-622-7937
www.mydna.com
www.webmd.com

Clinical Trials
American Cancer Society: 1-800-ACS-1234
Coalition of National Cancer Cooperative Groups:
877-520-4457 www.cancertrialshelp.org
National Cancer Institute (NCI): 800-4-CANCER
www.nci.nih.gov

Glossary

Abyss: An unfathomable chasm; an immeasurably profound depth or void, the abode of evil spirits; hell.

Acute: A sudden onset of symptoms or disease.

Acid Reflux Disease: See Gastroesophageal Reflux Disease.

Allergic Reaction: A response by the body to foreign material.

Anesthesia: Loss of feeling or sensation resulting from the use of certain drugs or gases. The use of anesthesia puts the person to "sleep."

Antibody: A substance produced by white blood cells in the body that helps to fight infection.

Barium: A white powder uses as a contrast medium in X-rays of the digestive tract.

Benign Tumor: Abnormal growth that is not a cancer. It cannot spread to other parts of the body. It can sometimes cause problems because of its location.

Biopsy: Removal and examination under the microscope of a piece of tissue from a patient.

Blood Cell Count: Number of red and white cells and platelets in a sample of blood.

Buccal Mucosa: Cheek lining.

Candidate: One who seems likely to gain a certain position or come to a certain fate.

Cancer: A general term for more than two hundred diseases characterized by abnormal and uncontrolled growth of cells. The mass, or tumor, can invade and destroy surrounding normal tissues. The cancer cells can spread through the blood or lymph system to start new cancers in other parts of the body. Also used to refer to a malignant tumor or cancerous tumor.

Caregiver: A person who helps and supports a patient through treatment and recovery.

Carcinoma: Cancer that begins in tissue that lines an organ or duct.

Catheter: A thin, flexible tube, used to place fluids in or remove fluids from the body, usually inserted into a vein in the forearm or hand (intravenous or IV).

CAT Scan, CT Scan, Computerized Axial Tomography: A sophisticated and accurate X-ray guided by a computer that looks at the body in cross section. For better contrast, a dye is injected into a vein. Sometimes an injection of dye into a vein is needed for better contrast. The process takes approximately thirty minutes to do one scan of one part of the body.

Cell: The individual unit that makes up all of the tissues of the body. All living things are made up of one or more cells.

Cellulitis: An infection of the skin that may spread to tissue just beneath the skin's surface. It may occur anywhere on the body, and is most common on the face or lower legs.

Chemotherapy: The use of chemicals (anticancer drugs) to kill or harm cancer cells and impede or stop the growth of a tumor; usually given as an injection directly into the blood through a vein. Also can be given in pill form and absorbed through the stomach into the bloodstream.

Concurrent Chemoradiotherapy: Chemotherapy given during the course of radiation.

Cisplatin: A chemotherapy drug widely used to treat more advanced head and neck cancers.

Clinical Trial: A study of drugs or procedures, conducted with volunteer human patients who are first to receive new treatments before they become widely available. The study may be carried out in a clinic or other medical facility; also called a clinical study.

Claustrophobia: A pathological disposition to feel terror in closed spaces; an abnormal fear of being in narrow or enclosed spaces.

Cure: When there is no evidence of cancer for five years—usually a fairly reliable time after which the chance of recurrence is extremely low. Some cancers, however, can be considered "cured" in one year while others cannot be "cured" even after five years. Each cancer is different.

Dehydration: Excessive loss of water from the body, increasing the need for fluids. Severe diarrhea or vomiting can cause dehydration.

Diagnosis: Name of an illness.

Dry Mouth (Xerostomia): Caused by lack of saliva in mouth; may begin a few weeks after radiation and may last for months or years.

Durable Power of Attorney: A legal document that lets you appoint someone to make health decisions for you if you become unable to do so for yourself.

Erbitux: (Cetuximab): A monoclonal antibody that works to bind and attack a specific structure on the surface of normal and tumor cells. Side effects are usually less severe than chemotherapy and radiation.

External Beam Radiation: A common form of radiation that directs a "beam" of radiation from outside the body, focusing directly on the cancerous internal organ and/or tissue. It may be used in conjunction with surgery, chemotherapy, and other treatments; uses a linear accelerator (high-energy X-ray machine) to direct radiation to the tumor. The procedure lasts a few minutes at a time, usually for five days a week, over six to eight weeks. Outpatient procedure.

Feeding Tube: A tube feeding is a method used to provide nourishment in a liquid form (special formula and/or water) into the stomach or intestine; the nourishment has the same protein, fat, carbohydrates, vitamins, minerals, and water as regular food. The liquid is dripped or pumped into the stomach or intestine by means of a tube in the stomach. Medicines may also be given through the tube.

GI: Gastrointestinal or gastroenterology.

Gastroesophageal Reflux Disease/Gastric Reflux: A condition in which stomach acid frequently backs up into the esophagus and throat. Over time cells may become irritated and change to create a premalignant condition.

Gastrostomy: Surgical placement of a feeding tube through the skin into the stomach for liquid feedings through the tube.

General Anesthesia: Drugs that cause a loss of feeling or awareness and put the person to sleep.

Gout: A type of arthritis caused by an unbalanced level of plebeian uric acid that strikes out of the blue, often at night, with excruciating, throbbing pain turning the skin red-hot and leaving the affected joint swollen and tender. It can last for days.

Head and Neck Cancers: A group of cancers that arise in the head or neck region (in the
nasal cavity, sinuses, lip, mouth, salivary glands, throat, or larynx).

Hospice: A program that provides palliative care and attends to the emotional, social, spiritual, and financial needs of terminally ill patients. Care can take place in an institutional setting or at home.

Hydration: Supplying water to a person in order to restore or maintain fluid balance.

Hyperventilate: To breathe fast or overbreathe. Anxiety is a common cause.

Immune System: White blood cells and antibodies that protect the body by attacking foreign substances.

Infection: Invasion by and multiplication of pathogenic microorganisms in a bodily part or tissue.

Infusion: Introduction of a solution into the body through a vein for therapeutic purposes.

Infusion Room: A room in a hospital specifically set up to care for patients in need of intravenous injections, blood transfusions, chemotherapy treatments, etc.

Injection: Using a syringe and needle to push fluids or drugs into the body.

Intravenous Injection: Using a syringe and needle to push fluids or drugs into a vein.

Intensity-Modulated Radiotherapy (IMRT): Highly modified beam of radiation that allows doctors to adjust the radiation dose more precisely to the tumor.

Intravenous/IV: Within a blood vessel.

Intravenous Infusion: A type of injection in which a drug, but not nutrition, is administered over a period of time directly into the bloodstream through a vein.

Isosource: A liquid formula made by Novartis that is high in calories and nutrients.

Kidneys: A pair of organs in the body that filter waste from the blood and excrete it as urine.

Living Will: A document that provides specific instructions about your health-care treatment.

Localized: Limited to the site of origin, with no evidence of spreading.

Lymph Nodes: Any of the small, oval or round bodies located along the lymphatic vessels, which supply lymphocytes to the bloodstream and remove bacteria and foreign particles from the lymph.

Lymph Node Dissection: A surgical procedure in which nodes are removed and examined to see whether they contain cancer; also called lymphadenectomy.

Malignant: Cancerous; has the potential to spread and invade other tissues in the body.

Metastatic/Metastasis: Cancer that has spread from its original site to other parts of the body.

Monoclonal Antibody Therapy: A new technique for treating cancer that involves very specific antibodies that will react specifically with the cancer cells. Side effects can be less severe than standard chemotherapy, but the technique has not been as widely proved to be as effective with all cancers and is still being tested.

MRI Scan, NMR Scan, Magnetic Resonance Imaging Scan: An imaging technique that uses a magnetic field and radio waves instead of X-rays to see structures within the body. The average time it takes is thirty minutes to one hour. Pictures are quite detailed. The patient must lie still in one position for the duration of the test. People with a tendency toward claustrophobia may feel anxious during the test. Medications can be given to help this anxiety.

Mucositis: Mouth sores that form as a result of cancer treatments, sometimes referred to as "ulcers" in the mouth.

Nutritionist: A health professional with special training in nutrition who can offer help with the choice of foods a person eats and drinks; also called a dietitian.

Oncologist: A doctor who specializes in treating patients with cancer, often the main caretaker of someone who has cancer and the one who coordinates treatment provided by other specialists.

Oncology: The branch of medicine devoted to the diagnosis and treatment of cancer.

Oncology Nurse: A nurse who specializes in caring for patients with cancer.

Oral Cavity Cancer/Oral Cancer: Types of head and neck cancer.

Oral Mucositis: Mouth sores caused by inflammation of the tissue lining the nose and throat.

Oropharynx: The area at the base of the tongue in the back of the mouth, including the tonsils. Cancer of the type that Dick has commonly starts in the cells that line the pharynx, and symptoms may include a sore throat that doesn't go away, trouble swallowing, a lump in the back of the mouth or throat, etc.

Outpatient: A patient who is treated but does not remain in the hospital.

Palliative Care: Treatment to relieve, rather than cure, symptoms caused by cancer. Palliative care helps people live more comfortably.

PEG Tube/Percutaneous Endoscopic Gastrostomy Tube: A soft rubber feeding tube measuring half an inch in diameter, that is inserted through the stomach wall during a brief operation under light anesthesia. If the cancer treatment is likely to cause the patient to be unable to take food orally, it is usually inserted before treatment starts and usually removed two to three months after the end of treatment. Used for nutritional support.

PET Scan: A more detailed scan to look at the cancer.

Pharmacist: A person trained in pharmacy; a druggist.

Phlegm: Thick, sticky, stringy mucus secreted by the mucous membrane of the respiratory tract, as during a cold or other respiratory infection.

PICC Line: Intravenous line that can stay inserted in a vein for up to six months.

Plain Radiography, Plain Film, X-ray: A standard X-ray of low-dose radiation exposure, which is generally painless or causes little discomfort. The average time it takes is one to five minutes.

Platelets: Special blood cells that help blood to clot.

Potassium: A mineral the body needs to maintain fluid balance and to perform other essential functions; an electrolyte in the blood.

Primary Tumor: The original tumor.

Primus: A type of linear accelerator machine used for radiation.

Prognosis: A doctor's prediction of how well a patient will do.

Protocol/VA Protocol: The plan for a course of medical treatment.

Radiation Oncologist: A doctor who specializes in using radiation to treat cancer and makes the decisions about a patient's treatment plan.

Radiologist: A doctor who specializes in reading and analyzing diagnostic X-rays, CAT scans, MRI scans, or other medical imaging.

Radiotherapy/Radiation Therapy: The use of directed radiation to harm or kill cancer cells. Radiation is used on tumors located in a specific part of the body. It can also harm normal cells; may be used alone or in combination with chemotherapy and other treatments.

Radiation Therapist: A person with special training to operate the equipment that delivers the radiation and who positions patient for treatment.

Radiation Therapy Nurse: A registered nurse who has extensive training in oncology and radiation therapy.

Recurrence: Reappearance of the same cancer after a period of time when there is no evidence of cancer.

Red Blood Cells: Cells that carry oxygen from the lungs to tissues throughout the body.

Remission: Partial or complete shrinkage of signs and symptoms of cancer.

Saliva: The watery mixture of secretions from the salivary and oral mucous glands that lubricates chewed food and moistens the oral walls. It contains ptyalin, which helps start the process of breaking down certain foods for digestion.

Salivary Glands: Secrete saliva and help digest food, prevent tooth decay, lubricate the tongue and throat for speech, and control bacteria.

Side Effect: An undesirable effect of a drug or treatment. All drugs have the potential to cause side effects. Common side effects of cancer treatments are fatigue, pain, nausea, vomiting, decreased blood cell counts, hair loss, and mouth sores.

Social Worker: A mental health professional with a degree in social work. A social worker can provide assistance in dealing with medical, psychological, social, and educational needs.

Squamous Cell Carcinomas: Malignant cancer tumors that develop in the tissues lining the hollow organs of the body. They make up 90 percent of oral cancers.

Squamous Cells: Flat cells that look like fish scales under a microscope. These cells cover internal and external surfaces of the body.

Stage: The extent of a cancer within the body, especially whether the disease has spread from the original site to other parts of the body.

> **Stage 1:** The cancer is limited to the tissue or organ of origin. The tumor is 2 cm (3/4 inch) or smaller (for head and neck cancers).
>
> **Stage 2:** There is limited, local spread of the tumor, which is about 2–4 cm; no spread to regional lymphatics, no distant spread.
>
> **Stage 3:** There is an extensive local and regional spread of the tumor but it has not spread distantly; with or without spread to lymph nodes. Its size is less than 6 mm.
>
> **Stage 4:** The cancer has spread (metastasized) to a distant part of the body or is larger than 6 mm or has invaded adjacent structures.

Staging: Performing exams and tests to determine the extent of the cancer and whether it has spread from its original site to another part of the body. It is important to know the stage of the disease in order to plan the best treatment.

> **TNM Staging:** Each of the following elements of a staging evaluation is categorized separately and classified with a number to yield the total stage.
>
> > **T = tumor:** T classifies the extent of the pri-

mary tumor, and is normally given as T0–T4.
T0 means that a tumor has not even started to
invade the local tissues. T4 represents a large
primary tumor that has probably invaded
other organs by direct extension, and that is
usually inoperable.

N = nymph nodes: N classifies the amount of
regional lymph node involvement (only
lymph nodes draining the area of the primary
tumor are considered). Distant involvement
would be classified as metastatic disease. N0
means no lymph node involvement, while N4
means extensive involvement. N2A means
metastasis in single lymph node more than 3
cm.

M = metastasis: M0 means no metastases (sec-
ondary tumors) and M1 means that there are
metastases.

A T1N1M0 classification means that the cancer is a T1
tumor, at stage N1 of lymph node involvement, and
with no distant metastases (M0).

Sonogram (Echogram/Sonograph/Ultrasonogram: An image,
as of an unborn fetus or an internal body organ, produced by
ultrasonography.

Surgeon: A doctor who removes or repairs a part of the body
by operation on the patient.

Tracheotomy: A new airway created through an opening in the
front of the neck. Air enters and leaves the windpipe (trachea) and
lungs through this opening. A tracheotomy tube (trake) keeps the
new airway open.

Throat Cancer: This is considered a type of head and neck cancer.
It is estimated that over sixty thousand people in the United States
are diagnosed with neck and head cancers each year, which represents about 5 percent of the cancers in the country.

Throat Cancer of the Oropharynx: A type of cancer that develops in the base of the tongue or in the soft palate of the back of the mouth.

Thyroid: A gland located beneath the voice box (larynx) that produces thyroid hormone. The thyroid helps regulate growth and metabolism.

Tissue: A group or layer of cells that are alike and that work together to perform a specific function.

Treatment Field: The place on the body at which the radiation beam is aimed.

Tumor: An abnormal growth of tissue that results from excessive cell division. Tumors perform no useful body function and can be malignant (cancerous) or benign (not cancerous).

Ulcer: A lesion of the skin or a mucous membrane such as the throat that is accompanied by the formation of pus and necrosis of surrounding tissue, usually resulting from inflammation or ischemia (restriction of blood supply to the area).

Ultrasound: A diagnostic imaging technique using sound waves to create an echo pattern that reveals the structure of organs and tissues.

White Blood Cells: Cells that fight infection.

Xerostomia: "Dry mouth" caused by radiation damage to the salivary glands.

X-ray: A type of high-energy radiation used to make pictures of the inside of the body. In high doses, X-rays are used to treat cancer.

About the Author

Gloria Burola McSorley is a mother of two and currently a grandmother of four. When time allows, she enjoys writing poetry, drawing, skiing, and taking walks in the mountains to find wildflowers. She grew up in New York, but after twenty-nine years she ended up in California. It was there her journey as a strong and extraordinary woman began, and later where she found her soul mate, Dick.

I watched my mother walk, willingly and without any reservation, the path through an unknown, dark abyss as she became Dick's caregiver from the moment he was diagnosed with cancer. She was an advocate for Dick while she put her needs and dreams on hold. Her life was transformed as she ate, slept, breathed, and felt every physical and emotional transformation with him. She experienced a little of what hell might be like, and in the end she became a person of great inspiration to those around her. It is her hope that through this work she can be a guide through those first one hundred days and nights for others who are about to embark on the life-changing journey of being the caregivers of cancer patients. Personally, I have learned from her to "look on the bright side" in my daily life, and it is my hope that I can become a woman of such strength if ever a situation is thrown at me that requires it.

— *Tammy Burola Blanchard, daughter*

ABOOKS

ALIVE Book Publishing and ALIVE Publishing Group
are imprints of Advanced Publishing LLC,
3200 A Danville Blvd., Suite 204, Alamo, California 94507

Telephone: 925.837.7303 Fax: 925.837.6951
www.alivebookpublishing.com